Yang-Style Taiji

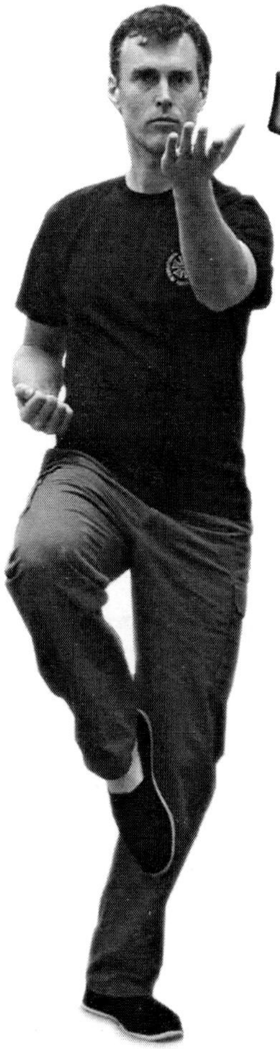

Yang-Style Taiji

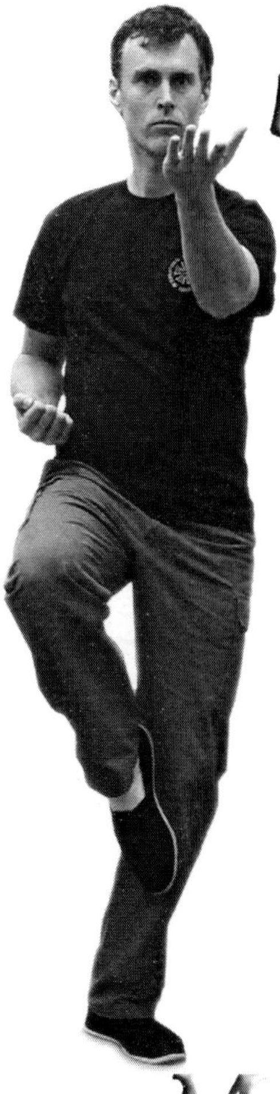

Michael Babin

Paladin Press, Boulder, CO

Other books by Michael Babin:
Power Taiji (with Erle Montaigue)
T'ai Chi Ch'uan: The Martial Side

Yang-Style Taiji
by Michael Babin

ISBN 10: 1-58160-618-4
ISBN 13: 978-1-58160-618-8
Printed in the United States of America

Published by Paladin Press, a division of
Paladin Enterprises, Inc.
Gunbarrel Tech Center
7077 Winchester Circle
Boulder, Colorado 80301 USA
+1.303.443.7250

Direct inquiries and/or orders to the above address.

Visit our Web site at www.paladin-press.com

Table of Contents

A Note on English Translations

For some years now, the official way of translating Chinese into English has been the Pinyin system preferred by the mainland Chinese government and accepted by a variety of international and academic associations.

Pinyin was first introduced in the early 1950s to replace the Wade-Giles and Yale systems of translation into English. You may come across spellings, not to mention misspellings and idiosyncrasies, from any of the three systems when reading books from different eras, sometimes even from the same era. Some examples of the variety of spellings are:

- Daoist was once "Taoist"
- Dantian was once "dan tien" and sometimes appeared as "dan-tien" or as "tan t'ien"
- Qi was once "chi" and sometimes appeared as "ch'i"
- Qigong was once "chi kung" and sometimes appeared as "chi-kung" or "ch'i-kung
- Qinna was once "chin na" and sometimes appeared as "ch'in-na"
- Taijiquan was once "tai chi chuan" and sometimes appeared as "t'ai chi ch'uan"
- Yijing was once "i-ching" or "i-ch'ing"

In general, I have used modern Pinyin spellings for place names but have retained the older, more commonly seen English spellings for proper names of the taiji personalities and the technical terminology of taijiquan. Consistency is nice, but so is paying tribute to "the old ways." There is a rich variety among Yang style taiji players that is mirrored in the written texts on that subject .

Acknowledgments

Good instructors are rare, but so are good students. In particular, Cal Climie, Michael Waterfield, and Alan Cumyn have been able senior students and teaching assistants to me in my ongoing Yang style classes in recent years.

I would like to thank them for posing for the photographs illustrating this book. I would like to thank Helen Kriemadis as well for being their very capable photographer.

My wife, Susan, and sons Marc and Eric have also shown remarkable patience with what must often seem like a quest on my part to prolong adolescence indefinitely.

Special thanks are due to my former Yang style taiji teachers; first Allan Weiss and then Erle Montaigue. If I have finally begun to understand what the Yang style can be like as an effective martial art, it was largely due to their instruction, example, and encouragement.

The other taiji instructors whom I have studied with or done workshops with since 1975: particularly Shirley and the late Steven Choi, William C.C. Chen, Carol Mancuso, Sam Masich, as well as the late Eric Chew have, each in their own way, helped me to understand greater or smaller pieces of the internal arts puzzle. However, any flaws in this text or in my teaching should be laid at my feet rather than attributed to any who have influenced me along the way in my development as a martial artist and taiji practitioner.

Finally, as a writer, I have a sense of humor and a moldering university degree in ancient and medieval studies in case you start wondering about the occasional bad pun or historical anecdote. You can contact me with your comments, questions, compliments, or complaints through the publisher or at my e-mail address: michael.babin@sympatico.ca

Foreword

by Allan Weiss

I feel most privileged to be asked to write a few introductory words for Mike Babin's new book. I first met him at the time that I began, with the approval of my own master, Lee Shiu Pak, to teach Yang taiji in Ottawa. Mike had already accumulated a significant background in that art from other instructors when he started coming to my classes.

It requires a certain humility, a dedication to excellence, a level of perseverance, and a determination to probe beneath the surface, to be willing to try other approaches that differ from what one has learned before—in effect, to become a beginner again—and Mike had all of those in spades. In the succeeding years, he has gone well beyond my own modest accomplishments. His book will be a welcome addition to the library of any serious practitioner of taiji.

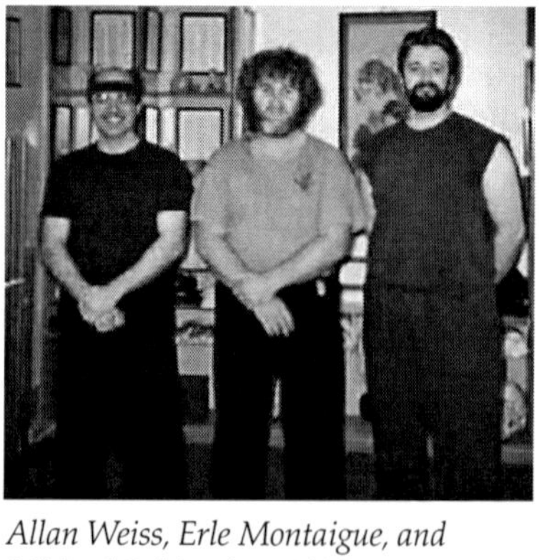

Allan Weiss, Erle Montaigue, and Michael Babin, circa 1990.

Foreword
by Erle Montaigue

I have known Michael Babin for many years as both student and friend. During that time, he has been one of my most promising students and, for many years, instructors in my system. His attention to detail is almost irritating! However, because of this, he has come to a very high level with his own training and teaching. This new book by Michael will prove to be of great value to any who should be brave enough to purchase it and read it. Brave? Yes, many will find that there are many aspects of this wonderful art that they are not aware of and which would only enhance their own training. Michael Babin is one of a few good men in this martial arts business, and I am happy that he calls me his friend. Good luck, mate; you deserve it!

Introduction

This book is aimed at those who have an interest in traditional Yang-style taijiquan. More specifically, it is written for those interested in both the health-building and meditative side of that discipline as well as the principles, tactics, and controversies of its martial side. (You wouldn't want to examine only one side of a costly antique coin before buying it from a dealer, would you?)

It is very difficult to find a complete curriculum in the Yang style, especially in North America, for a variety of reasons. These include a shortage of qualified teachers and the amount of time it takes to see results, which discourages many who start the training from continuing along that path.

If you are only interested in rebuilding your health or meditating, all you need is good instruction on a competent solo form. However, if you want to study the traditional martial aspects, then you need to find an instructor who knows the material, is willing to teach it honestly, and has the verbal skills to do so effectively. Not many that I have met fall into all three categories, which has lead to the decline of the Yang style as an effective martial system. This lack of comprehensive instruction has led to too many modern practitioners becoming content to study it in a superficial manner. As a result, in the past few decades the softer solo aspects of Yang style practice—the body (ti)—have been emphasized or divorced from the harder martial usage (yung).

The preservation and development of the art in North America has been further hindered as many of those currently teaching have not trained long enough with a competent teacher to have absorbed both sides of this taiji "coin."

Also, a considerable amount of New Age baggage has been used by naive or unscrupulous teachers to plug any gaps they may have in their own traditional training. In this way, the tendency among Westerners to look for meaning in their lives through cultures other than their own is often exploited by instructors, who have confused making money by wearing antique Chinese clothing and spouting pseudo-nonsense with developing real internal-style skills.

On the other hand, I am not suggesting that you need to become more Chinese than a native to be able to practice and benefit from your training. There is an unfortunate tendency in North American beginners to want or expect exotic and mystical results from their training. Perhaps too many of us have watched too many kung fu TV shows and movies while growing up.

Part of the overall maturation process for each practitioner is the result of correct methods done correctly! I have also largely excluded a detailed commentary on specific forms and training methods in anticipation of those who might be foolishly tempted to try to learn any such method exclusively from a text. In terms of physical movements and techniques, there really is NO substitute for hands-on instruction from a qualified teacher. Oh, and taijiquan should bring greater emotional peace and wisdom as the years go by, as well as physical skill and understanding.

I have tried to discuss the various issues covered in "plain English" whenever possible, as there seems to be a tendency in modern students to obscure such issues with foreign and esoteric terminology. Similarly, as there are much better texts available on the history of the Chinese martial arts and taijiquan, I have made little attempt to discuss this aspect in detail. Hopefully, those who buy this book may profit by reading my words even if it is only to stimulate their appetites to tell me just how wrong I am!

In the end, part of the overall learning process in any style of taijiquan—or in anything, for that matter—is deciding what your position is on various subjects and then being willing to alter those opinions, if such becomes necessary. I believe that it was the late Dr. Timothy Leary who, for all of his eccentricities, once suggested rather wisely that, "You are only as young as the last time you changed your mind."

Chapter 1
What is Taijiquan?

"Grand Ultimate Boxing" is the literal English translation of the Chinese characters used to represent *taijiquan*. While this certainly has a somewhat presumptuous sound in English, it is not a boast about the martial efficiency of the art, as is often assumed by casual readers. Instead, this term actually refers to *taiji*, which is a traditional Chinese philosophical concept about the interplay of the classic yin and yang energies. You can think of this relationship as being a way of expressing the idea that existence as we know it is really movement, rather than the apparent substance, as well as a constantly changing state of equilibrium within that movement.

The written character for yin originally literally represented the shady side of a hill and is associated with such qualities as darkness, cold, quiet, darkness, and femininity, among many others. Yang, by contrast, was the character used to depict the sunny side of a hill and implied brightness, heat, stimulation, activity, light, and masculinity, among other qualities. Everything is said to have both yin and yang qualities, and it is the interaction between these two forces that helps to create and maintain a healthy balance of qi in each individual as well as in life in general.

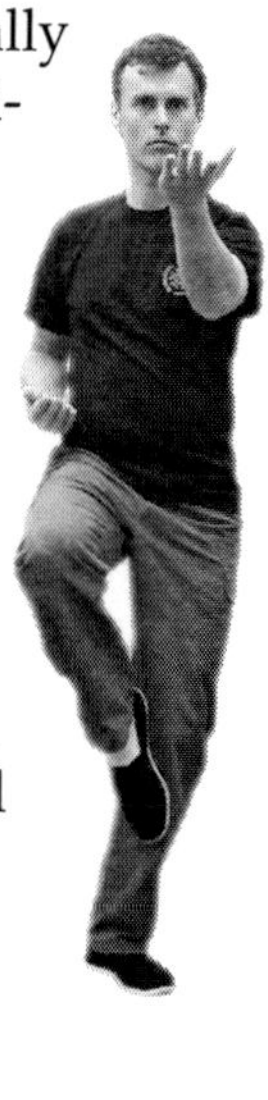

I have often thought (and have occasionally read in recent years) that a better English translation for "taijiquan" would be "yin and yang boxing," but that may sound a little too strange for many modern exponents who have gotten used to the traditional way of translation. Whatever label you use today, this discipline is many things to many people.

In a nutshell, learning taijiquan is about learning how to stand and move in a particular structurally sound manner while performing a variety of exercises by yourself and with a partner. This sounds easy until you actually try to copy movements and ways of holding yourself that are new to you, then add the challenge of doing so while training with someone else, as well as trying to heed the preferences of your particular teacher. Oh, and on top of that, the several different major styles of taijiquan all have slightly different ways of doing this!

Please remember that I am referring particularly to the Yang-style taijiquan when I say that this discipline can be:

- A means of relearning efficient physical posture and body mechanics while cultivating a stronger, more flexible, and balanced body as well as a calm and relaxed mind
- An introspective meditative solo practice that allows the individual to get in touch with him- or herself and accelerate the maturation process
- A martial art that specializes in close-range combat and includes means of striking, grappling, and throwing as well as tactics to counter these same tactics and is known for its use of neutralizing, yielding, and sensitivity skills as opposed to relying on brute force (as is often the case in the so-called hard style)
- A means of training to compete in a variety of regional, national, and international competitions by demonstrating excellence of solo form practice as well as mar-

tial sports excellence through push-hands and limited-contact sparring contests
- A means of exploring another culture by immersing one's self in the language and customs that gave birth to the art
- A fellowship that allows practitioners to meet and exchange information as well as foster friendships and relationships of many kinds, some beneficial and some exploitive
- A means for unscrupulous instructors to stroke their own egos while also making a great deal of money through exploiting the kind of blind obedience to a leader that many people seem to be looking for to fill an emotional void in their lives

To sum up, most modern teachers and practitioners will at least pay lip service to the idea that taijiquan is a form of exercise that can also be a form of meditation or a martial system for those with the interest. Not surprisingly, some of these criteria will overlap and some are apparently contradictory; but only the last is undesirable from a personal and social perspective.

THE HISTORY OF TAIJIQUAN

Much better historians than I have written in great detail about the historical context—and numerous controversies—of the development of the Chinese martial arts and of taijiquan and the Yang style. However, for those of you who have not done much reading on these topics, I offer the following brief history lesson.

Chinese culture and history is no different from any in the sense that, per human nature, being able to defend yourself was and is always an essential survival skill on a personal and a social level. Archaeological discoveries at the remarkable tomb of the first emperor of a unified China, many hundreds of years before the birth of Christ, have revealed dramatically how well organized and equipped the military and bureaucracy of the Chinese State was for its time. China was a literate society with well-developed cities, industry, and agriculture at a time when the ancestors of most Europeans were only starting up the long road to literacy and civilization.

In the 6th century AD, the Indian monk Bodhidharma (called Da Mo while living in China) came to the Shaolin Buddhist Monastery in Northern China. He is reputed to have developed a variety of calisthenics to improve the health of the monks, who seemed to him to be in sad physical condition from too much sitting meditation and too little physical activity. Over time these exercises were adapted into the martial arts that evolved from those practiced at the temple in his time.

Eventually, there rose a school of thought on martial training that took a fundamentally different approach. The legendary founder of taijiquan was a monk, Zhang San Feng, said to live in a Taoist monastery on Mount Wu Dang, who is reputed to have lived in the early days of the Manchu Dynasty (circa 15th century). Some scholars doubt his historical existence, viewing him as a literary construct on the lines of Lao Zhi, the supposed writer of the *Dao De Jing (Tao Te Ching)*, one of the seminal books of philosophical Taoism.

Others argue that Zhang San Feng was an actual person who linked the older martial practices with the meditative and medical theories of his time to create the fundamental thirteen postures of taiji (the famous eight actions and five directions still found in all family styles of taijiquan). Some report that the inspiration for his new system came while he dreamed about a struggle between a snake and a white crane; others say that his observation of such an actual fight was the inspiration. Whatever the inspiration, the exercises attributed to him stressed sensitivity and elasticity as opposed to the prevailing theory of using superior strength, speed, and technique to prevail aggressively in hand-to-hand fighting.

Closer to our time, Zhang San Feng's theories and practices were elaborated on by Wang Zhong Yue, who is reputed to have adapted the thirteen postures and linked them together, with repetitions and variations, into longer and more continuous solo sequences. His disciple, Jiang Fa, taught this system to the villagers of a town in Honan Province (most of whom had the surname Chen) and thus began the first—and oldest—family style of taijiquan. There are many contentious issues in taiji history and scholarship and some scholars feel that, rather than bringing an innovative martial system to the Chen village, Jiang Fa borrowed the essence of the martial system being practiced there, added it to what he already knew, and developed something of a hybrid.

In any case, the Chen village still exists and is still a hotbed of practice for this oldest existing style of taiji. In recent years, a variety of interpretations of that variation of taiji have appeared, but all trace their roots back to the source. Its practice is more obviously a martial art to the casual observer; the forms are done either slowly or at a faster pace with explosive movements, jumping kicks, deep stances, and well-rooted movements that emphasize twisting actions of the body and elbow strikes.

It is important to remember that the villagers had to practice methods that would be effective against brigands who might be wearing armor, in which case it made a great deal of sense to practice techniques that focused on controlling the joints (as this is always the weakest area in armor). This provides an unarmed fighter with the ability to throw an opponent down rather than futilely striking leather or metal armor with his hands.

This brings us to the last half of the 19th century when, for a variety of reasons, China was a land in turmoil. Western merchants, missionaries, and soldiers were entrenched in a number of important provinces and cities (including Hong Kong and Shanghai) and were anxious to exploit their technological and military superiority to secure advantageous trade agreements, as well as to control segments of the country itself.

This serious problem for the Chinese as a nation was compounded by the lack of any strong central government, as the corrupt and decaying Ching Dynasty seemed incapable of following the example that Japan had shown in the same time period in modernizing its industries, society, and government structure as a way of resisting the colonizing influences of the European and Western powers.

These larger issues, when combined with regional unrest on both a large and small scale, fostered social disorder in many areas. Once again, the more conscientious local Chinese magistrates and governors were obliged to repair the walls of their cities and towns as well as train and equip militias against an endless variety of bandits, revolutionaries, and human predators. In addition, floods, famines, and natural disasters seemed to come one after the other in rapid succession.

It was at this time that Yang Lu Chan became the first stranger in the Chen village to be allowed to learn their martial secrets. As with the story of Jiang Fa, there are many (often conflicting) stories of just how Yang came to learn the Chen style and later change it as he taught over the decades. Later in his life, Master Yang moved to the capital, Beijing, where he earned notoriety and considerable wealth through teaching a style of martial art that was based on the forms and methods that he had learned in the Chen village, as well as on his own experiences, creating what became increasingly known as the Yang style. I will describe the qualities of this style in greater detail in the next section.

Wu Jian Quan, a Manchu guard in the Imperial Palace at Beijing, was a student of both Yang Lu Chan and his son, Yang Pan Hou. Wu taught his art to (among others) his son, Wu Chien Chuan. From this stream of practice emerged the Wu style, which uses smaller and somewhat higher stances than either the Yang or Chen styles. It is most known for the significant forward lean in the postures found in bow stance, which is sometimes described as producing "ox-plowing power."

Chen Yau Pun was another Chen family member who abandoned what he had learned of the orthodox Chen style to create the "new" school of Chen-style taiji. His student, Chen Quin Ping, moved to the nearby village of Zhao Bao, and is usually credited as the originator of what is now called the Zhao Bao style of taiji.

In more recent years, Zhao Bao has been recognized as the sixth official family taiji style (the others being Chen, Yang, Wu, Hao, and Sun—each named after the founding families of the style). As another example of the controversies that plague taiji, either Zhao Bao is described as an offshoot of the Chen style, or the Chen style is contrarily described as an offshoot of the Zhao Bao style. The opinion will vary depending on to which camp the person to whom you are speaking adheres.

Wu Yu Xiang was a student of both Yang Lu Chan and Chen Qing Ping. Wu taught his nephew, Ly Yi Yu, who is often credited with having written one of the most important classics of taiji, *The Five Character Formula*. Ly and his brother were members of the upper middle class; this was unusual because at the time, the study of martial arts was denigrated as being suitable only for soldiers, security guards, and brigands. Some modern researchers believe that it was these two who actually invented the long two-person application set from the Yang style.

Ly, in turn, was the teacher of Hao Wei Zhen, who created his version of the Wu style, now usually called the Hao style. The Hao style is exceedingly rare today even in the country of its origin. It is unique in that it has very active footwork and relatively small stances as opposed to the larger, firmly rooted postures common in the beginner levels of all the other family styles.

One of Hao Wei Zhen's students was the famous xingyiquan and baguazhang master, Sun Lu Tang, who combined the essence of these three styles into the Sun-style taiji that he developed in his later years. Like the Hao style, his approach uses high stances and emphasizes mobility of the feet, but is perhaps closer, in terms of how it generates martial force, to xingyiquan. This should not be surprising, as xingyiquan was Master Sun's main art.

Master Sun's daughter and grandchildren continued to teach his arts in China, and in recent years the art has begun to spread to Europe and North America. Master Sun was of particular importance to the growing popularity of taijiquan in China. He was a scholar as well as a superb martial artist whose many published books popularized the idea that the internal styles were a family with roots in Taoism in the same way that the many hard styles had their roots in Buddhism and the Shaolin Temple. (Until Sun's time, the average Chinese practitioner, much less the public at large, would generally not have referred to any of the family styles as "taijiquan." That term wasn't popular until Sun started publishing his books in the period between the First and Second World Wars.)

Tumultuous times in China did not end with Sun Yat Sen's Democratic Revolution, the overthrow of the last Manchu Emperor, and the chaos of the Warlords Period that followed. World War II was a particularly terrible time for China thanks to the ruthlessness of the Japanese invasion. It is a bit of a paradox—but not a surprising one—that this was also a time of flowering for the martial arts.

In terms of the external styles, the various military colleges were encouraged to bring together various teachers and styles to study and simplify the traditional systems to produce effective styles that could be taught relatively quickly to soldiers. In the internal styles, teachers began to teach more publicly to aid in the process of strengthening the people and their will to survive, as opposed to the previous practice of limiting access to the arts to the strong and committed few. This was the time of the martial arts in general being referred to as *Kuoshu*, or National Arts.

By contrast, the post World War II Communist Revolution led to traditional internal and external arts being declared forbidden. Anyone who taught or practiced these styles were persecuted, and many old-style martial arts and qigong teachers went into hiding, taught only in secret, or left the country. During the infamous Cultural Revolution of the 1960s, the Red Guards even imprisoned or killed teachers and students of the traditional styles, as Chairman Mao felt that this training was part of the "old order" that was holding China back from making socialist and economic progress.

After Mao's death, the Chinese government gradually eased its prohibition against martial arts training, and a government-sanctioned style of sport-oriented martial arts (Wushu) was developed that emphasized the development of physical skills and solo competition. Until the 1980s, the Chinese government minimized the combative side of the traditional martial arts in an effort to make their citizens healthier—but not more liable to stand up for their rights; there have been too many revolts against government authority over the ages that were started by martial secret societies for the Chinese bureaucrats to encourage unrestricted martial training in the population.

More recently, the traditional martial arts have been "rehabilitated" and studied in depth. Many rare styles have been recorded and cataloged to preserve their history and practice. The original Shaolin Temple as well as the main monasteries on Wu Dang Mountain have been rebuilt or refurbished and their doors opened to foreign tourists of all kinds. Surviving older monks were allowed to return and young monks are being recruited and trained in both the old philosophical and martial practices. (I suppose that a cynic might point out that this may have more to do with cashing in on foreign dollars by martial arts tourists than a bureaucratic zeal to provide religious and martial excellence.)

Still, cynicism aside, thanks to easier immigration policies in recent years, many recent arrivals to Western countries are making aspects or whole systems from both traditional and modern versions of all the Chinese martial arts available more freely than ever before. In addition, the popular media worldwide has encouraged a renaissance in the combative sports so that more young people than ever before are training to compete in wrestling, boxing, judo, karate, and mixed martial arts events.

THE YANG STYLE

Whatever, the truth of the origins of the art, Yang Lu Chan was certainly a well-documented historical figure who passed on his considerable skill to his two sons, Shao Hou and Ban Hou. If half the stories about their training are true, Yang Lu Chan would certainly, in modern terms, qualify as a child abuser. However, it was a different time and a different culture, and both young men survived the training and, perhaps *because* of the severity of it, went on to became famous masters in their own rights.

Both sons, for a variety of reasons (perhaps due to their different body types and personalities) eventually taught their father's material slightly differently from him and from each other. Furthermore, they and their students after them would have been puzzled if you had said that the main reason for doing the art was to become healthy.

At that time, it was still primarily a fighting method, and you became a stronger, healthier person as a byproduct of your training; but that was not the primary reason that you took it up. However, despite its foundation as an effective martial art, even as early as the 1920s, some teachers were experimenting with modifying the art to make it less demanding and more accessible to larger numbers of people. For example, Yang Lu Chan's grandson and the son of Yang Jian Hou, Yang Cheng Fu, changed his father's form several times over the decades that he taught to try and meet the needs of larger and larger segments of the Chinese population.

This was also done, in part, to make the art more intellectually attractive to the middle and upper classes, who were prejudiced against the combative arts as being suitable only for ruffians and soldiers. Furthermore, China was torn by warfare between the various warlords and the central government, threatened by both Japanese and Russian territorial ambitions as well as Western economic dominance.

Over the many decades that he and his senior students taught in various cities in China, Cheng Fu took out the fast or difficult movements as well as the jumping kicks that had previously been part of the solo form and modified many of the training methods. He was responsible for both popularizing and standardizing the Yang slow form and curriculum. His style became the most widely known and practiced approach to taijiquan in China, despite the fact that he died at the rather young age of 53 in the early 1930s.

The oldest of Cheng Fu's four sons was Yang Sau Chung, who took his father's art to Hong Kong and taught it there until his death. He was among the many mainland taiji and kung fu masters who moved there shortly after the Second World War to escape Communist persecution. His tradition is continued by his oldest daughter, Mary Yang, as well as his three senior students (the late Ip Tai Tak in Hong Kong, Chu Gin Soon in North America, and Chu King Hung in Europe) and their respective children and senior students.

Cheng Fu's youngest son was Yang Zhen Duo, who was a preteen when his father died. Consequently, the young man learned most of his skill from his famous uncle and then from his late father's senior students, particularly Fu Zhong Wen. Zhen Duo's grandson, Yang Jun, has in recent years done much teaching for his grandfather around the world in workshops. He is being groomed to be the next head of the Yang family tradition.

Human nature and politics being what they are, some maintain that Yang Zhen Duo (being Yang Cheng Fu's son) is the leading light in the Yang family tradition, while others would give that distinction to the late Fu Zhong Wen and his son and grandson (because of the amount of time that Fu spent as Yang Cheng Fu's chief disciple and the young age and inexperience of Yang Zhen Duo when his famous father died).

Similarly, the descendants of the other famous senior students of Yang Cheng Fu—Chen Wei Ming and Tung Yin Chi—all state or imply that their version is at least as good, if not better, than that being taught by their peers in the Yang family lines of descent.

Although many instructors, both Chinese and non-Chinese, have claimed in recent years to do Yang Lu Chan's original form or that of one of his sons, there is no surviving evidence that any of those forms are identical to their supposed source. In some ways, though, falsifying lineage also seems to have been common in China, as venerable was always better and innovative martial approaches were always suspect.

Particularly, but not exclusively in the internal arts, there are a suspicious number of anonymous Taoist monks or mythical figures who are supposed to have transmitted their "secrets" in dreams or through mysterious texts that suddenly turn up when needed. I will elaborate on this issue in more detail in a later chapter.

Conversely, this doesn't mean that some of the modern versions are not closer to the source than others. For example, those taught by Erle Montaigue in Wales, Yang Jwing Ming and the late Kuo Lien Ying in the United States, as well as the late Chen Pan Ling in Taiwan, all had links to the older Shao Hou and Ban Hou sides of the family. Even though none of these versions have identical—or sometimes even similar—forms, their arts have a firmer, more martial aspect in both the forms and training methods than many other modern expressions of the Yang style that trace their origins to Yang Cheng-fu.

In the end, every teacher has his or her own version of taiji history and it is often impossible to sort out fact from fiction. In fact, I have given up trying to do so for the details of Yang-style history and am content to smile politely when someone insists on their version of history as being gospel—as long as the individual in question has something of value to share with his or her students and it is not a complete and obvious fabrication.

Similarly, there is a great deal of disagreement among the modern experts as to what is orthodox Yang style. Most divide the style into two broad categories: Yang family (the art as taught by the actual descendants of Yang Lu Chan) and Yang style (the art as taught by anyone who was a student of a teacher who was not a family member). Of course, there are those who consider themselves as teaching a family style because they married into the Yang family, but that doesn't always cut the mustard with Lu Chan's descendants.

Another major consideration is that those who have learned and taught the Yang-style taiji forms invented by the Sports Committees of the Chinese government also feel that what they teach is is at least as good, if not better, than that being taught by those who are more traditionally taught.

A cynic might also think that Cheng Fu and other taiji teachers who followed him simplified what they taught to the public in part to make it more acceptable to those wealthy enough to pay high fees for private classes, but whose temperament and physiques made it less likely that they would continue their training if they were subject to the rigor of the more traditional training. A few modern experts also believe that many of the prominent instructors in the 1920s conspired to conceal the most effective martial applications from those who were non-Chinese.

Since it started to spread to the non-Chinese populations in North America in the early '60s, taijiquan and, in particular, the Yang style were adopted first by the hippie and, more recently, the New Age movements, whose adherents believed through the translations and commentaries of a variety of American Buddhist writers and philosophers (notably, the late Alan Watts and the late Daisetzu Suzuki) that the softness and slow movement of taijiquan went well with the emerging ideals of nonviolence and ecological concern.

I don't mean to sound too touchy on the subject of "feel-good" taiji, as there is a real need for stress relief and environmental concern, but Groucho Marx was being intelligent as well as witty when he said, "I would never join any club that would have me as a member." Many modern taiji people seem to me to be exactly like that, but have banded together anyway in feel-good associations that have more to do with providing an atmosphere of mutual support than anything to do with quality training on any level—martial or otherwise.

This trend has been partially reversed in recent years by the immigration of a new influx of Chinese teachers and practitioners, as well as the proliferation of video instructional tapes and workshops with a variety of taijiquan experts. However, it remains true that it is easier to find mediocre instruction in taiji as a slow-motion dance than it is to find the real thing. Consequently, today most people think of slow, graceful movement, as in modern Yang style, as being the totality of taijiquan, as opposed to just *one* aspect of *one* style of traditional training.

As to a curriculum, if you want to study effective martial practice, look for a teacher who teaches you applications and basic fighting skills (entering, dealing with contact, and counterattacking almost at the same time as you yield or neutralize, etc.) as the groundwork to solo form training and push-hands.

As much as many people would like to believe otherwise, you cannot learn to defend yourself solely by being good at push-hands. Solo form cannot teach applications; it can only reinforce whatever you already know about effective interactive training. On the other hand, as it was in China, simplifying the art is due, in part, to the desire of some instructors to make the art more accessible to the elderly and the frail or handicapped. This is laudable in many ways ... as long as there are also competent, well-rounded teachers available for those whose health and interests take them in a more traditional direction as students.

Those who study my interpretation of the Yang style will be exposed to the following solo and partner training methods and forms. It will give you some idea of what is available in North American Yang style to compare my curriculum to that offered by your current or past teacher, or what to look for if you have not yet found an instructor or school that meets your needs.

Solo Training

- Three Circles Standing Qigong—This is a traditional standing-still meditation that generates and stores internal energy while strengthening the legs and teaching certain martial skills (particularly a whole-body usage of the arms and spine).

- Baduajin—This is a set of eight simple qigong exercises that can be used as a warm-up practice or done by themselves to strengthen as well as stretch the body while increasing the flow of internal energy to key areas. There are many existing variations of this set, and it comes in both hard and soft style versions. It is often taught by Yang style teachers as a supplement to the solo form practice.
- Yang Cheng Fu (long, slow) Form—This is the major solo sequence of smoothly connected and choreographed movement. This form is usually said to contain 108 individual postures or applications, partly because this creates the important number nine in Chinese numerology when the individual digits are added together. While this form can be executed at a variety of paces, it should take a minimum of 20 to a maximum of 45 minutes to perform once at a relatively even rhythm. It is practiced smoothly to circulate and balance the energy in the body while strengthening the legs and relaxing the upper body. It also reinforces the fundamentals of Yang-style taiji martial body mechanics.
- The Fast Applications Set—Erle Montaigue, whose version I practice and teach, calls this long, fast form *Paochui* or "cannon fist" form to differentiate it from the version of the same set done with a partner. However, this is not the same form with the same name that is practiced in some variations of the Chen-style taijiquan. In the Yang style, it is usually said to have 88 postures that are largely different from those found in the long, slow form. Practicing it solo allows you to train when you don't have a partner to train in the "fighting" side of it.
- The Short Staff Solo Set—This is a fast solo sequence using a 50-inch length of wood or rattan as a weapon. It is quite demanding physically and uses a large arse-

nal of techniques. I normally start intermediate levels of students with a simplified version of this set, as the full version takes a great deal of space to perform as well as strong legs and good taiji body-mechanics.

Training with a Partner

- Grounding and rooting—These are training methods that teach you proper body mechanics and posture within the context of learning to "stand your ground" and neutralize incoming force without doing so stiffly or just with the muscles of the arms and upper body. They also teach how to push and pull with the use of the spine and legs more than with the shoulders and arms.
- Uprooting—This is a method that trains a pair of students to relax and hold their ground while trying to push or pull their partner off-balance without having to move their own feet or lose their balance while doing so.
- *Tui-shou* or push-hands—These are training methods in sensitivity and yielding as well as other martial attributes and are designed to refine the ability of the student to use the four martial tactics found in grasp the bird's tail. These are half of the eight methods (*peng, lu, ji,* and *an*) that are the core of the Yang style as a martial system.
- *Da lu* or big pull-down—This is a formal method of practicing the other four main martial energies of taiji (*cai, lie, zhou,* and *kao*) as combined with stepping diagonally to the traditional five directions (*jin, tui, zuo gu, you pan,* and *zhong din*). It was said that it was necessary to learn da lu to compensate for any martial inadequacies that existed in your skill with tui-shou.
- Solo form applications—These are the martial usage of the individual martial postures found within the long, solo form. Training with a partner sharpens attacking

as well as defending skills. Striking a heavy bag or focus shields and mitts as well as controlled body contact are all aspects of such training.

- *Large san sau* is what Erle Montaigue calls the two-person method whereby you split the longer solo 88 Posture Fighting Form into two parts (A and B roles) and practice it so that both halves fit together like a martial puzzle. Practicing it with a partner is a way for two intermediate-level students to learn about distance and timing in a controlled manner that makes such practice relatively safe.
- *Chi sau* or "sticky hands"—This is a relatively unstructured version of push-hands that allows the practitioners to practice fighting interactions in relative safety because they are always in contact.
- *Fajing*—This is sudden, short-range expression of speed and power that uses the whole body to generate force and doesn't rely on arm and shoulder strength, or on having to retract the limb as a wind-up to the strike.
- *San sau* or free-fighting—This is the practice, with controlled contact to limited targets on your partner's body, of the ability to apply your martial skills in a spontaneous and unrehearsed manner. Doing so is the highest expression of timing and distance appreciation, as well as of yielding and neutralizing skills.
- Stick sparring—This is accomplished both through learning a simplified version of Erle Montaigue's two-person short stick applications form, as well as through practicing applications from the solo form and through a variety of conditioning exercises while using this weapon.

WHAT OTHERS TEACH THEIR STUDENTS

Other forms and training methods that show-up in competent versions of Yang family or Yang style taijiquan are:

- Variations on the unarmed partner-training exercises, particularly the sensitivity exercises that fall into the loose category of push-hands. Depending on the inclinations and training of the teacher, these can range the full martial spectrum that stretches from being overly genteel to overly brutal.
- Qigong methods from other Chinese martial or qigong systems that a particular teacher may have studied and has added to his taiji curriculum.
- Short solo and application sets that have been created by Chinese government Sports Colleges (e.g., the 24 posture form, the 16 posture sword set, the 48 posture combination form, folding fan and walking-stick solo forms) as an introduction to the longer and more demanding traditional sets, for competition purposes, or by individual teachers as a way of teaching "easy" taiji to the elderly or infirm.
- Broadsword (Yang style) and saber (Yang family) solo and application sets.
- Spear or long staff solo and two-person training methods. It is generally accepted that any long solo staff or training sets that may have existed in the Yang style are, for lack of a better word, "extinct." A number of such sequences are in circulation in recent years, but are relatively modern constructions (which certainly does not mean that they are worthless).
- Sword solo and interactive sets as well as a variety of training methods with that weapon.

NOW THAT YOU HAVE SEEN A COMPETENT MENU . . .

It has taken me many years to begin to come to terms with how to be a better teacher in the sense of simplifying the curriculum I make available in group classes, focusing on the core training methods, as this isn't an easy task to do without needlessly oversimplifying a curriculum. On the other hand, I have not yet come to terms with the lack of interest most students show by failing to attend the group classes regularly, much less how many of them fail to see the necessity for regular and committed solo practice on their own!

Sadly, the Yang style tends to attract students who often seem to get obsessed intellectually with the history and theory of the art. Perhaps it is easier to obsess about the past and search for "secrets" than it is to get up every morning and practice whatever you are trying to master. I have to admit that I spent years looking for the ideal teacher and "secrets" when I would have been better focusing on sweating over the basics. But that seemed so dull.

Of course, the reverse is also often true and I often meet practitioners who have no objective idea of the history and theory of their arts. They are content to swallow wholeheartedly whatever nonsense an unscrupulous instructor may want to feed them. *Caveat emptor* is not simply an empty phrase from a dead language!

In the next chapter, I will describe some of the ways in which you should approach the difficult task of being a competent student.

Chapter 2
The Learning Process

Once you have some idea of what you will be learning in a traditional Yang-style class, you have to find a good teacher. Fortunately, there are many competent teachers, both Chinese and non-Chinese, available now in North America. When I first started exploring taijiquan in the early 1970s, I had to learn my first taiji slow form from a book, and I don't recommend that learning curve to anyone, despite being an author myself!

However, getting the most out of your money, time, and effort isn't just a matter of finding a teacher; it is also a question of recognizing what you want from your taiji training as well as what you bring—both good and bad—to that training. Let's examine those first two issues before talking about what to look for in a teacher.

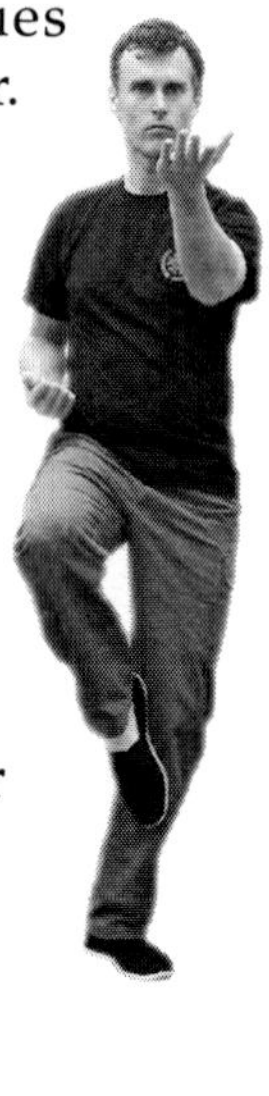

WHAT DO YOU WANT FROM YOUR TRAINING?

The first step is also the hardest in some ways, judging by the calls that I have gotten over the years from strangers inquiring about my beginner classes. Very few people seem to bother to do any research or even think through why they want to take classes before looking for an instructor.

The first few years that I taught, I was appalled by how often I asked prospective students why they wanted to try beginner-level classes, only to be told "I don't know," or "Your school location is convenient to where I work (or live)," or "My doctor told me to take it because I need to relax," or occasionally "I want to learn about an effortless way of defending myself."

Rather than going blindly into your classes, it might be more useful to consider the following issues when analyzing your motives and trying to match them up to your skills, weaknesses, and interests:

- Are you middle-aged or elderly, badly out of shape, or dealing with existing chronic medical problems? Are you looking for what you wrongly assume is a relatively easy and gentle form of exercise?
- Are you physically active and interested in learning martial forms and training methods that will challenge your fitness levels while bringing self-defense or competition skills?
- Are you too intellectual for your own good? Have you read books on Chinese culture, Daoism, or taijiquan that have interested you in the veneer of spirituality that has been imposed on this art in modern times?
- Are you intrigued by Chinese culture and hoping to broaden your cultural horizons or learn the language by interacting with members of that community?
- Are you bored and looking for something interesting to do one or two nights a week at your local community center?
- Are you hoping to meet a romantic or sexual partner through your classes, and is that more important than the quality of instruction in taiji that you receive?
- Are you looking for a master to provide guidance in your life and heal your troubles as well as a group of like-minded people to provide a support network?

It's tough to be honest with yourself about what you want from your training. You may discover with some reflection that you find a few, many, or all of these reasons for exploring taiji relevant to your needs.

It's also true that some of these are less desirable motivations than others, but beginners often start lessons for questionable reasons and learn to grow both as practitioners and as people through their training. Sometimes, the worst students in the beginning end up being those who "go the distance" and make progress that surprises the teacher as much as that individual. Sometimes, those who seem the best potential students are those whose interest burns out suddenly after a few weeks or months.

WHAT DO YOU BRING TO YOUR TRAINING?

A surprising number of modern students of the Yang style in particular, and the internal Chinese arts in general, have bought into the somewhat unusual idea that fitness is not only a non-issue in learning taijiquan, but that it is actually counterproductive to be fit when studying a traditional system! This is nonsense, although it is true that the Yang style can be practiced at a variety of levels and intensities by a wide range of students in terms of their relative age and fitness levels.

Your physical age is always relative to how well you have maintained yourself over the years, as well as to genetic factors. I have trained with 50- and 60-year-old practitioners who were fitter than many a modern 20-year-old. On the other hand, there is no doubt that the average older and previously sedentary students may have to modify the intensity of their efforts at first, coming to terms with their strengths and limitations as well as considering what personal and lifestyle changes will be necessary to train safely.

In athletic terms, we tend to peak in our late teens and early twenties and it can be a shock to realize that we are not as young as we once were. I have vivid and not overly pleasant memories of being told when I was in my mid-thirties that I would be classed as a "Senior" if I entered a particular taiji competition. The situation would be even worse now unless there was a Geritol Division!

In the long run, continuity of training is, of course, only possible if you practice a style that uses sound body mechanics. Allowing the knees to rotate out of alignment routinely, or repeatedly stressing the ankles, hips, or shoulders when practicing, may not seem to be a problem when you are young and fit, but in the long-run it may cause your joints to wear out prematurely when you hit 50.

This happened to me and I ended up needing a hip-replacement and, judging by many of the long-term martial artists that I know personally, such a fate is hardly unusual—although it is usually the knees, elbows, shoulders, and lower back that are the culprits. I will discuss this topic in more depth in a later chapter when exploring the issue of wear and tear from ongoing training.

Aside from being taught and then learning to use proper body mechanics, it is also important to practice moderately and on an ongoing basis. You may have to go on a diet or improve your fitness levels before beginning any interactive taiji classes, or pace yourself accordingly once you have begun to train, particularly if you have not led an active lifestyle or done any vigorous forms of martial training, no matter what your relative age.

One of the few good reasons for learning the long solo Yang-style form first, as is often done nowadays, is that practicing this sequence competently can begin to restore physical health to those who were not previously active in anticipation of that student later being strong enough to do the martial training safely and effectively.

Of course, with proper stretching and progressive training, any martial ability can be gained to a surprising extent even by the older beginner. However, he or she will have to be prepared to train more carefully and moderately than the younger students in the class. Human nature being what it is, it can be very difficult to restrain yourself when everyone else around you seems to be moving faster and working harder than you!

If you are practicing the fast forms and are past 35 years of age, I recommend taking one day off every week from martial training. However, standing qigong or slow form should be done every day or at the very least on alternating days. Older beginners should consult with a physician before beginning classes in even the slow form of Yang style taijiquan, much less the martial activities, especially if they are seriously overweight, unused to physical activity, or suffering from chronic medical conditions.

In some ways, it is no longer politically correct to speak of aptitude in the sense of some people being naturally more talented than others in their individual learning curve, but it is difficult to ignore that this is also often patently true. In the end, the students, no matter what their relative aptitudes or ages, are only at a real disadvantage if they try to exceed their capabilities or rush their progress.

Evaluate Your Attitudes

Becoming competent at any aspect of the Yang style is not simply a process having a good teacher or of mastering how to stand and move your body while doing a form or training method. It is also often a process of relearning the learning process. This can be particularly difficult for those adults who have settled into a hectic lifestyle that no longer includes a sense of fun or acquiring new habits. While you certainly can teach an old dog the proverbial new trick, it is equally true that this is much harder to do when the old dog has lost the habit of playing, much less learning.

There's a price to pay for everything and your leisure time is usually curtailed to some degree if you become serious about your training. This may be fine if you're single, but it may cause problems if you're not. For example, your girlfriend may not understand why her dinner party seems less important than your scheduled workshop, or your husband may not understand your sudden desire to attend classes three times a week and may worry that it will interfere with the family routine.

Studying any aspect of taijiquan can mean doing what you think is right for you even if others don't immediately understand or support your interest. However, as few of us are reclusive monks living in a mountain cave, we also have to remember the need for compromise. One of my best teachers, Erle Montaigue, has often said, "You should do taiji to live; not live to do taiji."

Many beginners take up the Yang style because they have been told by health professionals that such practice will help them to learn how to reduce their stress levels. Unfortunately, judging by my conversations over the years with doctors and nurses, most have usually never done any style of taiji. Similarly, many students interpret this promise of relaxation to somehow mean that they will experience relief just by attending classes.

The ugly reality of having to work hard, pay attention, and take corrections after a long day at work or at college is more than many can bear. I once had a lady approach me at the end of her very first introductory class to say that she would not be returning. She wasn't going to pay me to correct her efforts in class, she said, as she had enough corrections from her boss at work every day.

It is difficult to pay attention at the best of times, and it can be particularly difficult when you have to add new physical skills to the intellectual side of the art. This can be especially hard for modern people who are bombarded by information at a breakneck pace in advertising, television, and movies. "Taking your time" seems increasingly to mean that you only do two or three things simultaneously instead of multitasking as many activities as possible.

So don't be surprised if the first few months of classes serve only to elevate your stress levels when you discover that taiji is not as effortless as it can look. It is no longer surprising to me that many beginners stop training almost immediately when they find out how demanding of their time and effort the Yang style can be. I'm not necessarily talking here about the martial classes either, but the relatively easy qigong and slow motion solo forms that most beginners are looking for.

In addition, few students are prepared for the length of time that it will take to learn a long, traditional sequence of postures. This reluctance is one of the reasons that so many short, simplified sequences have been created in recent years to try and coax beginners into continuing to train. Many are shocked to learn that taiji was and can still be a great martial system. Even those who have heard of push-hands may be discouraged from trying the martial side when they learn that there is a risk of injury in such training and that not everything is done in slow motion.

Perhaps the greatest stumbling block for the average American student is his or her lack of both patience and a realistic understanding of what learning taijiquan should be like. Even with adequate and sincere instruction, a novice is more likely to leave class tense and frustrated, especially if that individual is unhealthy or unused to regular physical activity.

Set Realistic Goals

A minority of gifted students, no matter what their age, will have one intuitive breakthrough after another in their training. However, most of us will only create a deeper understanding of ourselves and our taijiquan one element at a time, over the years. The following five strategies may help you make the most of your training and avoid injury:

1. Set progressive and realistic goals and put them in writing. Reassess and change your goals at regular intervals as you train over the months and years.
2. Keep a daily training diary, even on those days that you don't train. Studying the reasons that you didn't practice on a given day may help you determine how to break bad patterns and counterproductive habits.
3. Expect setbacks. There may be minor or serious injuries that require a period of rest and rehabilitation. You may be away on business or have family commitments that take precedence temporarily with your training. Long-term, moderate effort is the ultimate key to being able to train for the rest of your life.
4. Don't be too proud. Keep your skills and accomplishments in perspective and identify those areas in your training that still need work and can be improved realistically.
5. Don't be too humble. Mastering a difficult aspect of your training should be acknowledged with pride while you continue to remember about step number four! It is also wise to remember that a good instructor can share what he or she knows with you and can correct your efforts, but that he or she cannot do the actual work for you. If you don't practice, then you are wasting both your time as well as your teacher's, not to mention the money you have paid in fees.

THE ROLE OF THE TEACHER

As a beginner, it is always preferable to have the best possible instruction, as it is easier to create good habits than to correct bad ones. However, it is also sadly true that good instructors are almost as rare as good students and that everyone has to start somewhere.

In any case, the average beginner will probably not be able to do more than crudely copy an instructor's movements, whether those are of high or low quality. Despite this, it is not always easy to find any instructor, much less a good one, unless you live in a big city where there is more likely to be at least some choice of potential schools of taijiquan. Where do you start?

- Search the Internet or phone directory for schools and teachers in your area. I should point out that it may be difficult to find very good instruction in taiji if it is being taught as a sideline activity at a commercial martial arts school where the main focus is in the Japanese, Korean, or Chinese hard styles. It is also true that there are always exceptions to this cautionary note and you might be lucky in who you find.
- Look through the flyers or Web sites of any continuing adult education programs in your area or at your local community center to find entry-level taiji in the "for-health" category.
- If you are a college or university student, check to see if there is a club on campus that can provide affordable entry-level instruction. The instructors in such venues are often foreign students who may have learned a great deal in China, Hong Kong, or Taiwan despite being relatively young.
- Visit the local parks that are used by the Chinese community in the early morning, and try to find groups of people practicing taiji together. To be honest, it is sometimes hard to be accepted by such a group, whether or not you are Chinese, but a friendly smile and a willingness to try are sometimes the best ways into such a learning environment.

In the end, the best way of finding competent instruction is to talk to friends or coworkers already involved in taijiquan or in the martial arts. Good word-of-mouth is the best form of advertising there is for any competent teacher and the one who is usually the most trustworthy for beginners.

Once you have found someone to learn from, you need to be careful about putting him or her up on a pedestal. There are always instructors willing right from the start of their teaching careers to be worshipped by their students. Others start off with good intentions but are slowly seduced into thinking of themselves as special because of the hero worship they receive. My father once expressed this with rather crude eloquence when we were discussing human nature as, "If enough people line up to kiss your butt, you have to be pretty smart not to eventually start thinking that there's something special about it!"

Some instructors tread the fringes of exploitation by misrepresenting just how internal their skills are when they are really skilled only in a hard style and teach one or two taiji forms as a sideline. Many of the latter will teach a taiji form that they learned at a workshop or from a video as a way of expanding their potential pool of students, even though they are not much further ahead in skill level than their students.

Some otherwise talented instructors tread the fringes of exploitation by forcing their senior students to teach beginners' classes for free. This is a traditional approach to getting help in coaching beginners in larger group classes and, in all fairness, can be a valuable learning experience for the more experienced students. On the other hand, the more experienced students may not know how to teach yet, which shortchanges the beginners with less experience and aptitude. Conversely, the time spent with novices cheats the experienced students if they spend all of their class time teaching instead of practicing with each other or the instructor.

Another way some instructors tread the fringes of exploitation is by having grading systems that call for frequent and expensive tests. (By the way, color sash systems are still relatively rare in Chinese systems, but are becoming common in the more commercial martial arts schools, as they are a great way to raise revenue for the teacher or operator.) In this way, the monthly fees may seem affordable, but you have to factor in the charges that you will have to pay every few months for yet another grading test.

Still another way some instructors tread the fringes of exploitation is by playing head games as a way of testing the loyalty of their students, either to see how much they can exploit them, or to see how hard they are willing to work. To be fair, though, it's also true that many teachers don't consciously do this, but are reflecting the way they were raised or trained.

A few teachers have no problem with ethics, as they dispense with them altogether and take advantage of their students fairly openly. Although money or egotism are usually the culprits, the sexual urge is also a potential pitfall that traps many. When the Yang style was in its infancy, there wasn't a problem caused by mixed classes—as there weren't any. Women learned only from their husbands or fathers, and only if there was a need to teach them (e.g., they lived in a dangerous area when the menfolk were not always available to defend the home, or there were no sons available to inherit the system).

Even into the 20th century in China between the two world wars, women experts sometimes taught middle and upper-class women form and qigong, but rarely the combative aspects of the art and never in mixed classes. While this was sexist in Western terms, it also avoided contentious issues that often come up in modern classes, such as those men and women who are looking for relationships more than quality taiji, as well as those men who feel that they can fondle female students under the pretense of having accidentally made contact during the martial training.

It is also true that, at least for the first few years, the student—no matter what his or her gender—who wishes to learn deeply needs the instructor more than the instructor needs students. Any teacher tends to attract and retain like-minded students and vice versa, which is one more reason for having or developing some common sense and a little self knowledge before attaching yourself to your chosen role model. One of my senior students once said to me, "Have you ever noticed that all your long-term serious students are just like you—independent and grumpy eccentrics?" I think he meant it at as compliment.

One of the most difficult aspects of finding a good teacher is that many decent practitioners are not particularly good teachers because they don't have the patience, the language, or the communication skills (and, no, the last two items are not the same thing).

I don't speak or read Chinese and for many years didn't think that it mattered in terms of doing a decent interpretation of taijiquan. Now I'm not so sure anymore. Part of the problem for non-Chinese learners lies in their Chinese teachers having poor English language skills in terms of explaining the finer details of practice to their students or being able to answer questions in their second language. Of course, it is equally true that immigrant Chinese will have the same problem in reverse with native-born North Americans who may be experts in taijiquan and speak only English, Spanish, or French.

Oh, and on the subject of languages, it is common enough to find non-Chinese teachers who have adopted a Chinese "professional" name for a variety of reasons, primarily to appear more knowledgeable. To make the issue more confusing, sometimes good non-Chinese practitioners are bestowed Chinese names by their Chinese teachers, partly as a mark of distinction and partly because the Chinese name will be easier for the Chinese teacher to say than the English pronunciation!

On the other hand, a good instructor is not necessarily someone who speaks Chinese fluently (at least to your ears!), has a nifty uniform, or who can do a seemingly endless variety of solo forms or push you crudely off-balance while doing push-hands because he is 40 pounds heavier than you. It is also true that appearances can be deceiving. Sometimes those individuals who look initially like anything but martial artists can surprise you with both their personal skill and their teaching ability.

I once had someone that I was doing push-hands with at a "free-play zone" between various clubs say to me, "You don't look like you can do anything, and yet I can't affect your balance no matter how hard I try." I took it as compliment, although I don't think he meant it that way.

On the other hand, it is easy to get burned out even when you come to teaching with the best of intentions. For example, when I first started teaching in 1985, I was full of grand intentions. Twenty-plus years later, my attitudes toward teaching have somewhat hardened and I have acquired a great deal of sympathy for those old-timers who refused to spoon-feed students who expected to get handed all the answers just because they had paid their fees and showed up to class on time.

This is not to say that instructors and their students must be saintly and free of human error, although many students seem to expect their instructors to be this way. Nor am I suggesting that the average student should kowtow to a prospective instructor, shower him or her with presents, and hang around his or her front door day and night until accepted as a student. Such may have been appropriate in another time, another culture, but it's not so appropriate today.

As a student, you owe your instructor the respect and courtesy you expect to receive from him or her, combined with patience and effort to learn the skills being offered. If you decide to stay with a particular teacher for the long term, you owe that individual a measure of loyalty. This kind of martial loyalty implies an honest and mutual exchange, and the willingness on your part to trust the instructor's motives and skills without losing sight of the fact that he or she is human.

Traditionally, you were expected to undergo a taiji apprenticeship of many years before beginning to teach on your own. Often this would happen only when your teacher died or retired. Nowadays, many instructors are teaching after only one or two years of instruction. Even with the proper foundations, a new instructor will take some time to come into his or her full stride, even with all the proper foundation of skills and a clear understanding of how to teach the material. Sadly, some novice teachers will never get much better, no matter how many years they teach.

Of course, it was a also little easier in the good old days to know if an instructor had skill at least on some martial level. The other martial artists and instructors would visit and offer, politely or otherwise, to beat the &^%*# out of him. It's difficult to fake competence in a martial art when a stranger is doing his best to throttle you.

It is also true that many instructors rise to a certain level of competence (or incompetence) and then never change no matter how many years they continue to practice and teach. It seems to be human nature to believe that you know it all and changing your approach to taiji is not easy, especially if you do have some skill and have had good instructors. One of my former senior students said it best when describing what one of his teachers of the automotive mechanics craft had said to him: "Do you want to be someone who has learned for 20 years, or someone who has done a year's work 20 times?"

In the end, you have to learn to teach yourself many of life's lessons, but a good teacher can certainly make that learning curve a little easier—if not painless. The only way to find out if a particular teacher, or the Yang style in general, is compatible with your talents and needs is to follow him or her long and well enough to see if you benefit from the training.

This, in turn, implies that you develop enough skill to judge for yourself. Whoops, that becomes a conundrum along the lines of, "Which came first, the chicken or the egg?" when you are trying to decide which teachers are bad, adequate, or excellent. This is not an easy process, particularly for beginners.

Of course, such confusion is also an essential part of the learning curve if you are serious about your training. I was discussing the very issue with one of my fellow instructors and this person was moaning and groaning about how hard it is to teach properly and how little enthusiasm or skill that the average student brings to this discipline. I suppose that the old masters were muttering the same thing 150 years ago in the Chen village and 75 years ago in Shanghai and Beijing, when the Yang style was at its height as a martial system.

In the end, a good teacher eventually makes him or herself redundant by teaching each serious student how to continue to evolve without his or her guidance. It is similar to parenting in that a competent parent works at ensuring that his or her children develop the necessary skills to face the world on their own. Perhaps this was originally part of the the idea in the Chinese concept of a martial student treating his teacher as an adopted father.

A good teacher should be an expert in what he or she is teaching (both theoretically and practically) before he or she begins to do so. Conversely, it is equally true that teaching can make a good practitioner and teacher even better with time. Of course, this also implies that the students you teach down the road a decade or two will get better instruction than those you taught at the beginning of your career.

But, if it's of any consolation to those who realize that they were "early students" of a particular teacher, I'm sure that even though Stradiavari was producing even more superb violins at the end of his career, the ones he made in his first few years were probably still pretty damn good. Everyone has to start somewhere on every journey.

FINAL THOUGHTS ON LEARNING

Finding a teacher is rarely easy, even if you live in a big city where there are most likely at least some resources available. In addition, a good style may only have poor representatives in your area, or a sterling example of a style may be your first fleeting contact with it and then every other representative that you meet subsequently is a bitter disappointment.

There's an old Chinese expression that states that learning taiji is a lot like putting money in the bank: Make a small deposit every day and you will reap the interest, but only much later in life. In this way, regular and ongoing practice on your own is an essential supplement to regular attendance at group classes. Don't be like the woman who once asked me in all seriousness at the end of a 10-week introductory session that I had taught at a community center, if it would have been a good idea to practice between classes. I'm not often at a loss for words, but that was one such occasion.

Once you have found a good teacher who suits your needs and abilities, train with him or her until you have squeezed that person dry of information and have to find another, even better teacher—or when can stand on your own two feet as a seasoned practitioner (but this is not usually the matter of a few months or even years).

In the next two chapters, I will discuss, in some detail, standing qigong and the long, slow form, as these are both pivotal basic methods for both the self-healing and martial sides of the Yang style. Training without solo forms makes it difficult to understand the health-building and meditative side of the Chinese internal arts. Focusing solely on techniques and sparring, however, can make you a great fighter, but is liable to ruin your body as you get older and does less for the "spiritual" side of your training.

Chapter 3
Core Methods:
Standing Qigong/Standing Like a Post

I would hope that the average student would realize after a few lessons with any competent teacher that it is important to create a coherent structure to truly benefit from one's taijiquan practice. Building a house can be a useful analogy, as with both pursuits one must certainly follow certain steps in the correct sequence. If you buy a piece of swampland, get the order of construction wrong, or use faulty materials, it is difficult to avoid having a house that looks like it was constructed by amateurs. It's always good to know your limitations and respect them by sticking to what you do well. This applies equally to taijiquan.

In the context of this discipline, doing things in the correct order implies that a student will learn how to breathe naturally and relax unnecessary tension, and will learn or improve efficient posture and sound body mechanics, strengthening his or her mind and spirit. Ideally, all of this will be well on its way before he or she begins to work on the martial side of the art.

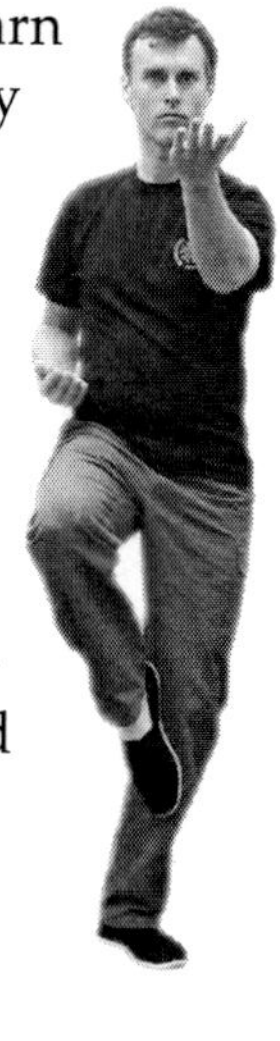

Indeed, many students will never willingly go beyond this initial level and will remain content with the varied benefits (improved flexibility, greater leg strength, improved eye-hand coordination, and more relaxed and straighter posture) that certainly may be gained from the solo training, without ever once touching another person in a martial sense.

Getting started properly requires two fundamental aspects to your solo training: standing meditation and long, slow form training. Most beginners have some idea that taiji involves moving the body slowly in specific ways, but very few are familiar with the concept of standing or sitting still as being an essential aspect of learning the art. It's not surprising that this is so, as not many modern teachers are familiar with the practice. Many of those have given up trying to use it in their general classes.

Most students who come to class to learn the slow, graceful movements that they have seen elderly Chinese doing in parks don't want to be told that standing still for long periods of time is beneficial—even essential—to such training.

Most North Americans can't envision sitting still for a few minutes, much less standing still and appearing to do nothing for five or even 15–30 minutes at a time.

Conversely, a few will find themselves strangely attracted to standing qigong and will practice it excessively while neglecting the movement aspects of taijiquan (more on the pitfalls of this later in the chapter).

If you are going to learn to be still and to move in a Yang-style manner, then it is important to have at least a simplified understanding from a traditional perspective of why you would want to do this. This implies talking about what the Chinese call internal energy, or *qi*. Having some familiarity with the relevant terminology is also valuable in terms of understanding some of the cultural traditions associated with the cultivation of qi.

On the other hand, getting obsessed with such terminology and theory becomes less valuable if you apply the products of your research too literally to your training or meditation. In general, the modern teachers who talk the most specifically about this internal energy and how to approach its cultivation in a variety of extreme ways are those who strike me as being exploitive rather than beneficial to their students.

The term *qigong* means, literally, "breath or energy work." It is a relatively new term, having been coined in China in the 1950s to describe the exercises that were based on the traditional methods known as *neigong* (which referred to exercises done to strengthen the body in different ways while also cultivating particular states of mental and spiritual well-being).

This tradition of practicing methods to strengthen and heal the body, mind, and spirit can be traced partly through oral tradition as well as through archaeological discoveries of artwork and written texts going back at least to the Chinese Bronze Age, thousands of years before the birth of Christ. Judging by the evidence now available, even at such an early time, calisthenics of various types (perhaps in the form of ritual dances) were taught both as a means of religious celebration and as a means of warding off or curing a variety of chronic illnesses.

In later centuries, the yogic traditions came to China from the Indian subcontinent with Buddhist missionaries and traders. These systems were to blend with native traditions and have survived and thrived in their Chinese forms, despite centuries of warfare, social upheaval, and the occasional persecution by Confucians and Communists alike.

While much intellectual baggage has been overlaid onto traditional practices in the last hundred years, first to make it more attractive to the Chinese educated classes and then, much later on, for middle-class Westerners, it is not strictly essential to believe or even understand any such theory to benefit from the physical practice. Similarly, for those with strong Christian or other religious feelings, there is no need to embrace any Chinese religion to be a successful practitioner of qigong. However, in my experience, many middle-class North American exponents will go to the opposite extreme and try to become more Chinese than the Chinese practitioners of old! Contrary to what I often see among my peers, you don't have to wear an ancient outfit or fancy uniform, learn to speak or read Mandarin, or spout pseudo-oriental wisdom to benefit from your training—in fact, usually it is an impediment to progress. In Japanese Zen Buddhism, the tendency to get caught up in the external trappings rather than the principles of your practice has been referred to as "stinking of the Buddha." In my experience, the same thing could be said of many of those Westerners who study qigong and Daoism.

Conversely, we do live in a more conservative age, and a surprising number of clerics seem to feel that their flock may be tainted spiritually by practicing qigong or taijiquan. More than once over the last decade, I have read articles by fundamentalist Christians and Muslims alike denouncing taiji or qigong as being the tools of Satan. Sadly, tolerance and religious zeal rarely seem to go hand in hand. For those of a religious conservative bent, this is one more issue with which you will have to wrestle in your search for tools to improve your physical health and broaden your well-being.

However, It is also true that even a superficial understanding of Daoism and Chinese culture can be relevant to those who choose to study qigong. When contemplating this, it is also important to realize that there are a number of types of, for example, Daoism. That word can encompass:

- The philosophical musings of Lao Zhi (Lao Tzu) and Zhuang Zi (Chuang Tzu)

- The Five Elements and yin/yang theories that are the underpinnings of Traditional Chinese Medicine (TCM)
- Sexual tantric practices ("dual cultivation")
- The rituals of a popular religion with shamanistic roots and a complicated pantheon of gods, spirits, and immortals

As with the European alchemists of the Middle Ages, some Daoists also indulged in an obsession with transmuting metals and herbs into formulae which, it was hoped, would bring immortality to those taking them. Unfortunately, experimentation with toxic metals (mercury and lead in particular) brought insanity or shortened the lives of many—including at least one Daoist emperor—and eventually led to most abandoning the search for a literal pill. Instead, the emphasis shifted to using breathing and visualization techniques to search for spiritual, if not physical, immortality to produce the same results without toxic side effects in the present life.

AN OVERVIEW OF QIGONG THEORY

Qi is indefinable, although the Chinese, like the Inuit of Canada's Far North who have many words for the various qualities of snow, have many words for the different qualities of that concept.

In more traditional terms, practicing any method of qigong is about creating, storing, and maintaining an optimal amount of internal energy as well as refining and circulating it throughout the body for a variety of purposes. There are several categories of traditional Chinese qigong: self-healing, martial, medical, and spiritual. In turn, these can be from a Daoist or Buddhist (and even Muslim) perspective; however, there has been much blending over the centuries and many methods cannot be neatly pegged into one category.

There are two major categories of qigong: passive and active, although, again, there can be a crossover in that some methods of passive qigong do involve slow movements of parts of the body. In traditional terms, practicing any competent method of qigong for health maintenance is said to be "good for the qi," whose energetic circulatory system of 20 main energy lines transports this vital force to every cell of the body. While the qi is said to lead the blood, the latter is said, in turn, to support and nourish the qi.

Of these 20 lines, there are 12 channels as well as eight vessels. The former are each connected to major organs or regulate organic processes; the latter are storage reservoirs and major conduits for internal energy. Two of the latter are particularly important: the Governing Vessel, which starts at the bottom of the torso and goes up the spine and over the top of the head to the upper palate, and the Conceptor Vessel, which begins at the tip of the tongue and runs down the center of the front of the body to the bottom of the torso.

In addition to these, there are also countless unnamed minor channels which, like blood capillaries, carry qi to every cell of the body and are said to nourish the bone marrow—which is a major player in both traditional martial meditative practices as well as, in modern terms, the immune system. These minor channels also connect to the pores of the skin on the surface of the body.

Any physical or emotional injuries, as well as muscular tension, can impede or block the smooth and balanced flow of internal energy within the body and to the surface of the body, affecting the health in various ways. Fortunately, imbalances will often clear up on their own, as qi always seeks to balance itself. In addition, qigong doctors are said to be able to affect this energy system beneficially in a variety of ways: the use of acupuncture to affect energy flow by inserting needles into the appropriate acupuncture points, the application of different forms of massage, herbs applied to the skin as well as burned over the skin at strategic locations or taken internally as medicine, and the application of the healer's energy through what is called "distance healing," which a Westerner might think of as the older practices of the "laying on of hands" in faith healing.

Various methods of self-healing qigong can also be used to improve and maintain health by ensuring a normal production of this energy and to refine its quality as well as open and balance energy circulation throughout the body. It is important to remember that the TCM approach was very different from Western medicine in that one of its major goals was to prevent illness from taking hold, rather than focusing on curing problems that spring up from bad living habits.

As a beginner, don't worry about harming yourself by practicing any basic standing qigong method incorrectly. You can't create an illness or disorder through faulty practice, although you certainly can waste your time or suffer minor physical discomfort (e.g., muscle strain, sore joints) from faulty or lackadaisical training. This assumes that you are a "normal" person to begin with and not in the acute phase of a serious physical or mental illness. If you are, you should consult a qualified qigong doctor and only practice under his or her supervision.

There is hardly unanimous agreement on the value of standing qigong. Going by my personal experience over the years with a variety of teachers, it is quite interesting to compare samplings of some the different attitudes to standing qigong that I have encountered:

- It is completely unnecessary to do any standing-still qigong, as the slow form and the martial forms and two-person training provide everything you need.

- You don't need to learn solo forms or martial training of any kind. Just stand properly and your health and martial skills will be superhuman after many years of doing just this, as long as you practice for hours each day, every day.
- You must follow a "secret" progression of standing methods that go from simple to very complex.
- Pick a posture at random from the slow form and practice it on both sides while gradually increasing the amount of time that you stand until you are doing so for at least an hour each day.
- Use the initial/final posture of the long, slow form as your basic standing qigong practice and do it *before* your daily practice of the slow form.
- Use the preparatory posture of the long, slow form as your basic standing qigong practice and do it *after* your daily practice of the slow form.
- Use the initial/final posture of the long, slow form as your basic standing qigong practice and do both before *and* after your daily practice of the slow form.
- Only practice simple standing methods that don't strain the joints. Even five minutes per session is enough if you do that regularly and pay attention for every second of the five minutes.
- The method must involve deeply bending the knees or standing on one leg at a time and must exercise the strength and stamina of the arms by holding them in complicated postures so that you learn a new kind of strength.
- Use elaborate visualizations of the micro- and macrocosmic circulation and do them only under supervision, as you can harm yourself in energy terms and go crazy.
- Don't use elaborate visualizations. Stand quietly, simply smile, and relax the mind and body as much as possible.

- You must learn to breathe in an essential sequence of methods (e.g., deep abdominal breathing; followed by Daoist reverse breathing, followed by tortoise breathing).
- Don't pay attention to your breathing in any way, except to ensure that you refrain from holding the breath.

If you persevere in your standing training, you will eventually find the approach that suits and seems to benefit you and, perhaps someday, you will even be able to have a chuckle or two over the confusion that you put yourself through in the early years!

It is also interesting to note that some traditional taijiquan experts have argued that their arts are not forms of self-healing qigong, as they are too martial. I do agree with those who feel that the Yang long, slow form—at the very least—certainly falls within that category in both physical and energetic terms.

Many teachers demonstrate a variety of self-healing qigong, both standing and sitting. This is done to broaden the suitability of their classes to a larger audience as well as to reflect the varied interests and experience of a particular teacher. In Asia, it was and is still common to find martial arts and taiji teachers who were also good practitioners of at least one aspect of TCM. In North America, this is much less common, although it is interesting to note that some teachers who hold doctorates unrelated to any healing arts, Eastern or Western, will often insist on being referred to as "doctor," perhaps because of this tradition in the Far East.

Incidentally, martial qigong methods (e.g., Iron Shirt and Qi Packing methods) can also be good for you, but tend to be more physically demanding and harder to practice safely and correctly from a technical point of view. I'll touch on the subject of martial qigong in a later chapter.

You can divide the development of qigong into four basic categories, although again, there can be overlap in the purposes of some such exercises. For example, methods that are self-healing can obviously have relevance to martial training qigong in the same way that medical qigong is often associated with those who practice the more spiritual methods as well:

1. Self-healing methods are designed to allow those who practice them to strengthen their health and resistance to disease or to cure an existing illness or medical condition.
2. Martial training methods are designed to strengthen and train the body and will of the practitioner to resist being struck and to develop skills that will support the practice of the traditional Chinese fighting arts.
3. Medical methods are designed to strengthen the internal energy of the qigong doctor or healer and aid him or her in treating clients with a "hands-on" application of qi as a supplement to the other means of treating illness from a traditional perspective (e.g., acupuncture, acupressure, massage, and the application of herbal poultices, soups, and pills).
4. Spiritual methods are designed to help the practitioner become a more highly evolved person in meditative or religious terms.

These categories often blend and overlap, depending on the bias and training of the person teaching you, and can be accomplished from a Daoist, Confucian, Buddhist (and even Muslim or Tibetan) perspective. However, there has been much blending over the centuries and many methods cannot be neatly pegged into one category. In turn, the methods themselves can be done lying down, sitting, or while standing, without moving or while moving.

Meditation

Lying Down Methods

There are many statues and paintings, both ancient and modern, of the Buddha and various Daoist immortals that depict them doing this style of meditation while lying on one side with eyes closed and pillowing the head with one bent arm. Such methods are often prescribed for the elderly or those suffering from serious illness or who lack the physical ability to stand or sit for long periods of time.

Lying down qigong can also be very useful for any beginner in terms of learning basic muscle relaxation skills as well as practicing more advanced methods of visualization and meditation. Unfortunately, one of the major drawbacks for practitioners at any level of experience is the ease with which one can fall asleep while lying down with your eyes closed or partially closed. In fact, my wife has even accused me of stretching the truth when I assure her that my lying on the living room couch on a Sunday afternoon is actually qigong training.

Sitting Methods

Sitting methods are most often associated with the more demanding spiritual meditative practices, as they can be done for longer periods of time without excessively fatiguing the body and with eyes closed to minimize the lure of the senses when practicing. As with the first method, falling asleep can be a problem for practitioners. In some traditions of group sitting meditation, it is common to have one monk or practitioner whose duty it is to walk quietly among the meditators with a stick and hit them firmly on the shoulders if they look as if they are starting to drift from meditation into slumber.

I have been told more than once by teachers over the years that standing practices are best suited to the relatively young for health building and martial training, while sitting practices are best suited to those older practitioners who are focusing on spiritual meditative training. However, I'm not sure that this is necessarily so, as sitting cross-legged in the Buddhist manner is quite painful for most Western practitioners initially. While it can contribute to increased flexibility in the lower body, it can also aggravate existing troubles with the joints in older beginners.

In fact, some of the more extreme sitting positions in the Japanese and Indian traditions can be needlessly hard on the joints of older Western beginners who are not used to sitting in such positions. Fortunately for Western practitioners, who are more used to sitting in chairs, Chinese traditional qigong methods of this sort are often taught while sitting in relative comfort on a chair or bench with both feet naturally and comfortably on the floor. On the other hand, the practitioner is also often told to sit up straight without using the backrest on the chair or bench so that the spine benefits from having to "sit tall." This can take some getting used to for Westerners unused to doing anything but slumping in an office chair or sofa.

Standing Methods

I will be focusing on standing still and moving qigong, as that has been the primary focus of my training over the decades. Such practices involve a wide spectrum of possible activities, ranging from standing almost perfectly still for longer periods of time, to standing relatively still in terms of footwork, while using movement of the arms or torso and while using the mind for visualization of energy movement in the body, or while breathing in particular patterns.

I recommend standing practices to anyone who is serious about their Yang style studies on any level. In this way, those interested in improving and maintaining their health should do this practice to complement their study of the long, slow form. Standing still is said to generate and store energy as its main (yang) activity, while it circulates and balances energy flow throughout the body as its minor (yin) activity. The long, slow form in terms of vital energy does the reverse of this, so you can see that both methods are necessary for balanced long-term practice. Those interested in the martial side of the Yang style should do standing still qigong for at least one year—if not longer.

Some teachers tend to force their students to do this right from the beginning of the training, partially as a way of weeding out the insincere or faint-hearted students. Other teachers will wait until a student has demonstrated considerable skill and loyalty before revealing this "secret" training method. Still other teachers will talk about it and introduce it at random and then wait to see who among the student body shows an interest. Oh, and some teachers give up with modern students and just ignore the subject of standing still training all together.

The Three Treasures

Compared to the complexities of the long, slow Yang form, standing qigong methods minimize the physical aspects of training (in comparison to the more complex moving forms) so that it is easier to concentrate on what is called "regulating the three treasures"—the body, breath, and mind.

Body

Even though the physical body doesn't seem to do much work aside from holding itself up in a relatively still fashion, it is actually relearning muscle usage and body mechanics so that the spine is stretched, relaxed, and energized to easily and efficiently support the head and internal organs. The legs and hips are loosened and strengthened while the knees relearn to transmit the weight of the torso efficiently downward to the ankles and feet. Your knees are not designed to be weight-bearing, although they are often given that task though bad postural habits (e.g., knees that sag habitually either outward or inward) or uneven muscle development in the legs.

In addition, standing meditation is not as comfortable as sitting meditation, so you must concentrate on the appropriate amount of muscle relaxation in order to do the exercise with increasing ease. In this way, the entire body learns to use only the right amount of tension in the muscles to keep the body comfortably upright and balanced. The torso and arms must, in particular, be relaxed and feel connected to the feet. In turn, this brings a sense of whole-body connection that is so important to doing taijiquan properly.

As the joints and body loosen, the internal energy is better able to circulate internally. Think of it as your internal energy circulating through hoses that are often partially impeded by kinks of varying degrees—like a garden hose that has become knotted or crushed. The energy inside cannot flow easily until these kinks are removed.

As standing becomes more natural for you, as the lungs expand and the joints relax, circulation improves, often lowering mild hypertension and preventing or alleviating conditions like varicose veins and hemorrhoids. Even if you practice correctly, your legs and lower back may get quite sore at first, but this is normal, especially if you are tense by nature or not used to regular exercise.

By the way, it is easier to learn deep relaxation while lying down, as the muscles don't have to do ANY work to hold you up. You are also more likely to fall asleep rather than meditate. In the end, a standing posture trains the body in functional relaxation and this means there is less chance of getting drowsy. Similarly, keeping the eyes at least partially open is also done in part to reduce the chance of falling asleep and collapsing.

Breath

There is a short phrase often attributed to the late father of modern Yang style, Yang Cheng-fu, that reminds us that our breathing should be, in general, "long and deep, fine and even."

"Long" refers to encouraging each breath to be full and relatively slow, but without obsessing about or forcing the breath, as doing so is always considered inappropriate by the better teachers.

"Deep" refers to encouraging each long breath to start in the lower torso and to feel as if it fills and empties the entire torso—not just the chest area. An interesting analogy that can help you get this idea is to imagine that you have a long straw that reaches from the nose down into the lower torso/lower dantian. When you inhale, the lower area relaxes and expands, pulling the air in and down; when you exhale, that upward and outward movement of air is powered by the contraction of the muscles of the lower torso.

"Fine" refers to encouraging each long and deep breath to be smooth and noiseless so that you are not huffing and puffing or gulping air in your attempts to improve the function of the lungs.

"Even" refers to ensuring that a long, deep, and fine breath has roughly the same amount of time in the inhale and exhale phases of each breath.

Breathing this way is equated to relearning the way in which a young child breathes before growing old enough to copy all of his or her parents' bad physical habits. This reeducation should be a gentle and long-term process. In this way, you retrain the diaphragm to rise and fall over a greater range so that the lungs are used more efficiently. This augments the capacity of the lungs, while the greater range of movement in the diaphragm also produces a massaging effect on the internal organs, thus improving the functions of the digestive, reproductive, urinary, and endocrine systems.

Don't try to keep your chest from moving even though you want the breathing to feel as if it is centered in the lower torso. It is important to remember that sinking the breath and the qi to the lower dantian does not mean forcing the lungs to overinflate, nor does it mean swallowing air. You are not a puffer fish, so don't act like one!

By the way, it is quite common, as a beginner, to get quite "gassy" when practicing—so don't get too embarrassed in class if you belch or pass wind. Over the months, your digestive system will adjust and this won't be as much of a problem. (There is a persistent story among experienced practitioners that the best way to find a new teacher to practice with in a park is to find the area that smells the worst, as it means that the new students are actually having their internal workings stimulated and not just practicing movements of the arms and legs!)

Breathing abdominally is essential for several reasons. It retrains the diaphragm to participate fully in making the breath deep, full, and even. The in-and-out movement of the lower torso actually strengthens and loosens the abdominal and psoas muscles (without having to do sit-ups) so that you are less likely to have back problems caused by weakness. In traditional terms, the lower dantian should act as a qi pump to spread energy easily throughout the body. Abdominal breathing is essential to make this happen most efficiently.

Don't force the breathing in any way. That includes trying too hard to use abdominal breathing. The breathing should be encouraged to deepen and slow down, but don't try to force yourself to breathe correctly, as causing tension through trying to improve breathing is hardly a worthwhile approach to learning how to relax.

One last note on breathing: I know for myself that the best sessions of standing qigong for me have a rising and a falling quality that starts in the heels, rises through the head, and falls back into the heels. The Daoist sage, Lao Zhi, wrote, "The true men of old breathed through their heels." That sentence never made sense until I started experiencing it in qigong. Some qigong experts maintain that rocking the weight gently and rhythmically forward and back or keeping the toes curled under lightly activates the Bubbling Well acupuncture point (yongquan/kidney #1) on the bottom of the foot, which is the key to accessing earth energy.

Of course, in a structural sense, it is essential that the body weight stay on the heels (rear part of the foot) most of the time. If the weight stays forward on the ball of the foot or the toes, it can raise too much yang energy and cause what is sometimes called "adverse cyclical qi." In pragmatic terms, keeping your weight too far forward or too far back on the heels for long periods of time means that your weight won't be falling efficiently through your knees. This can lead you to injure them with regular standing, especially if you are overdoing the amount of time in each session and not balancing that training out with an equal amount of movement exercise.

Mind

Although it it's difficult to do, the conscious mind must be encouraged to give up its obsession with endless mental activity. The Chinese refer to this overactive mind as a "monkey," because it's always scampering about being noisy and causing trouble.

However, quieting unnecessary mental activity does not also mean that you go into a trance, hypnotize yourself, leave your body, communicate with spirits, or try to become some form of superhuman. More realistic and desirable goals include learning to focus the mind on fewer and fewer distractions so that eventually you can stand and simply be attentive and connected to "what is."

Qigong students are often told to visualize elaborate circuits of movement of energy when they practice, as doing so is a simple form of biofeedback that promotes relaxation. Without relaxation, stressful thoughts can heighten blood pressure, lower certain hormone levels, elevate others (adrenaline), and weaken your efforts to build better health.

One school of thought on this subject believes that since modern research has demonstrated that biofeedback can be effective as a method of metabolic regulation, the physical processes describe as happening during qigong can only be aided by imagining a microcosmic orbit or similar meditation. Conversely, performing this exercise without such visualization can only bring about lesser results.

As far as I am concerned, I agree with those experts who feel that the ultimate goal of standing qigong as mediation is to quiet or empty the conscious mind and that elaborate mental "games" or visualizations can cause additional mental tension when the practice should be minimizing, if not eliminating, that very mental tension! However, simpler visualizations or mental exercises (e.g., counting the breath or repeating a healing phrase) can act as an essential stopgap to learning about the sung state.

Some authorities insist that the qi must rise up the front and down the back, while others insist just as vehemently that it naturally rises up the back and down the front. Others insist that you should be able to control it at will, depending on the martial or meditative process. I have always felt that it is best not to try to consciously control or interfere with whatever normal flow of energy exists in the body. In fact, these days I tend to explain qi to my students as being a form of biochemical electricity or a motivating spark. This may make us sound a bit too much like an automobile, but it seems a valid comparison in many ways.

There are several ways to start relaxing the mind and focusing it in desirable ways:

- Count each slow, gentle exhalation while paying attention to the physical movement of expansion and contraction in the lower abdomen.
- Create your own short healing phrase (e.g., "This calms and heals in every way") and repeat that silently to yourself in time with each breath. I suggest that you time the length of the sentence so that a relatively slow inhale of five seconds and a relatively slow exhale of the same length is necessary to repeat it once to yourself.
- Be aware of the feeling of being connected to the earth through the soles of the feet while using peripheral vision (an unfocused gazing of the eyes) to be attentive of everything around you while listening passively to the sounds of your environment. This is another way of being "present," though detached, mentally.

STANDING LIKE A POST (ZHANGZHONG)

Those Yang-style teachers who still teach standing like a post sometimes use a wide variety of methods and sometimes focus solely on using the beginning posture of the long, slow form as their basic or sole such method. For those who are unfamiliar with this practice, I will describe it in some detail, as these details are common to most basic methods of standing qigong.

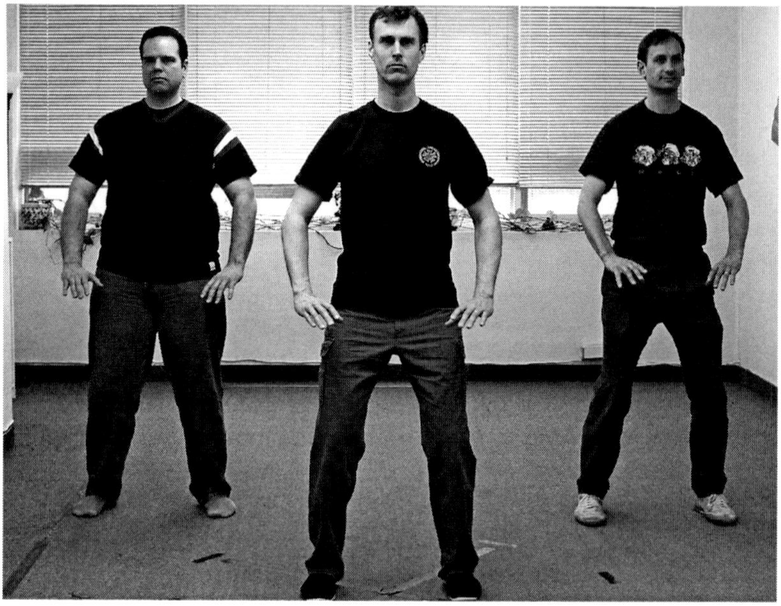

Left to Right: Mike, Cal, and Alan stand still holding the preparatory/concluding posture of the Yang long form, which can also be used for standing like a post training, either before or after the practice of that traditional sequence.

POSTURAL GUIDELINES FOR STANDING

- Begin by stepping to the left with the left foot if you are male and to the right with the right foot if you are female. Your feet should end up about the width of your hips apart and you will bend your knees slightly until the knees are roughly in line with the toe tips. Hold your palms facing down near the outside of your hips with the elbows gently bent and the feeling of holding a small apple in place in each armpit with the pressure of the upper arms.
- Have a gentle lifting feeling from the top of the back of your skull, as if you were gently suspended from that point and your head and torso were hanging comfortably downward. This feeling is very different from simply stiffening your neck and sticking your chin out in

too "military" a manner—for lack of a better word—nor should it look as if you are slumping. Perhaps it will help if you get the image of your body being like that of a marionette being held in place by a skilled puppeteer. In any case, you want a feeling of gentle expansiveness throughout the spine and head.

- Keep your forehead smooth and free of furrows of concentration and your eyes open slightly, so that you look far forward and slightly downward at the "big picture" in front of you.
- Inhale and exhale quietly through the nose. Keep your teeth and lips closed. Put a slight smile on your face; smiling in this way can actually aid in releasing muscle tension in the jaw and face.
- Keep your neck straight and comfortable, especially where it connects to the skull.
- Relax your shoulders, with the scapula pulled somewhat together and encouraged to drop slightly downward.
- Let your arms feel heavy yet relaxed; allow your elbows to curve slightly; keep your palms pressed downward with your hands turned slightly inward.
- Keep your spine long and relaxed, as if every vertebrae were pulling gently away from its neighbor above and below it.
- Allow your sternum to be empty, as if you have just sighed. Doing this frees the ribs, heart, and lungs to move as they should.
- Relax your abdomen. Let it expand as you inhale and compress as you exhale. Think of this process as relaxing, not forcing, the abdomen and use some muscular force when contracting the muscles of the lower torso.
- Relax your tailbone so that your pelvis and the lower spine between the kidneys is able to move as freely as nature intended it to do.

- Keep your crotch open and rounded as if you were sitting on a pony. Distribute the weight evenly between both legs.
- Lightly close and lift your perineum. In general terms, you should always try to maintain a gentle lifting feeling in the crotch, as this serves several important functions. The gentle "squeezing" or "lifting" feeling is essential in activating the "energy pumping" function of the lower dantian. It gently tones the muscles in the pelvic region. (Never exaggerate this use of the muscles, as you can give yourself a hernia if there is weakness in that area.) In traditional terms, it also closes the anal area to encourage the upward flow of energy in the governing vessel as well as minimizing "qi leakage" out the anus.
- Keep your legs as relaxed as possible and your knees bent to the correct angle for the entire time that you practice. One way to learn how this crucial leg angle feels is to stand facing a wall while placing the tips of the toes gently against the baseboard and then bending the knees until the kneecaps make contact with the wall. Close your eyes so you don't get flustered by having the wall "in your face" and get someone to watch you stand for a few minutes to give you feedback on whether you are leaning forward or backward or putting more weight on one leg than another; both of these are no-nos in your standing practice. Don't press too hard with your toes or knees, but be able to tell if your knees lose contact with the wall as they straighten.
- Let your feet "sink" gently into the ground or floor, weight dropping into the center of the sole. You should have a feeling of being rooted and connected to the earth and not just sitting on its surface.

For the first weeks after you start such training, you will probably only be able to remember all of the details of correct posture when you are obsessing about them, or correcting yourself with the help of a full-length mirror or a friend who is watching you practice and offering you feedback.

In fact, for the initial months that you stand regularly, you will not be doing much in terms of mental relaxation or "quiet," as there is too much too think about in terms of details of posture, not to mention the discomfort of standing itself. Reviewing the postures mentally in the sequence given here as you begin your practice on a particular day can help you relax the overly tense parts of the body as you pass through them on your way downward. A useful way to do this is to record yourself reading the postural requirements on an audio tape and play it each time you start your training, until you don't need such audio cues anymore.

Once you have stood for the length of time that is appropriate for you, you can finish with some gentle exercises, walk around a little, or do the long, slow form.

General Guidelines for Standing Health

One of the most important guidelines that I can offer you is to get competent instruction, at the very least for your initial training. It is very difficult to learn anything that can be practiced both safely and meaningfully through self-instruction alone. Sadly, we live in an age of quick fixes and general impatience—many modern students are loath to do anything more demanding of their time and money than buying an instructional book or video. There are many such products and some are very good indeed, but they may be of use to you only after you have some relevant skill and experience.

In addition, having some experience in yoga or having learned Buddhist sitting meditation or Reiki at a weekend workshop doesn't automatically make it easy for you to learn how to do any competent method of standing qigong.

For most of us, "pride goes before the fall," and it is easy to overestimate the value of your previous experiences when learning something new. This seems especially true among those who have bought into the New Age concept of qigong as being both a physically easy and spiritually esoteric way of training.

For those who are reading this and already study with a competent teacher, don't be surprised if he or she disagrees with some of the details of the following guidelines. My comments are based on my own long-term experience as a teacher; they are not just comments repeated mindlessly because my teacher said it was so or because I learned superficially from a video or textbook.

Although some teachers, both of the traditional and New Age persuasions have come up with an amazing number of rules in relation to qigong, I feel that there are relatively few important issues to keep in mind.

Where, When, and How Long Should You Practice?

Whenever possible, train outside in a natural setting near running water or among trees. This is particularly true in the springtime. Some traditionalists would say that you should never practice indoors, but must train where your feet are in contact with natural soil and your body is surrounded by the outside air with the sun above you. Even in winter, it is a good idea to practice outside, although you should take care to train in a sheltered area, particularly in relation to strong, damp winds. If you must practice indoors because of the weather, try to do it in front of a window (especially if you have a view of nature) or on the balcony of your apartment if you have some privacy and shelter from rain and wind.

Conversely, a few experts that I have met say that practicing indoors is best, as the "good qi" will accumulate in that location and create a beneficial place for you to train.

(See how easy it is to sort out the truth when researching any aspect of taiji or qigong!)

Daily practice of both standing and moving mediation is preferable and ideally will be done in the early morning or early evening. In the good old days, this meant literally at sunrise and sundown. As those times change with the seasons, it could be quite challenging to follow such a schedule when you have a family and work obligations and are not getting up with the chickens! For example, some experts advocate that the best time for standing qigong and long, slow form training is when the Lung Meridian is most active, which happens to be between the hours of 3 and 5 A.M. This may not fit into your daily schedule.

If, like most of us, your daily life is rather hectic, try alternating your practice in the sense that you do standing qigong one day and then the long, slow form the next, and so on. If you are practicing the martial aspects of taiji, then you could alternate doing the health-building methods one day and the martial solo training on the next day.

As far as I am concerned, the ideal is to be in accordance with the natural rhythm of the day (i.e., more active in the morning and day, less active in the evening and at night). There is a wide variety of opinions on this subject, however, and in the long run, it is essential to find a time of day that you can practice with some regularity rather than skip practicing because you can't fit it into the ideal time.

I tell my students that they are fooling themselves if they train in an irregular manner. In his translation of the book on Sun-style taijiquan by the late famous internal master, Sun Lu Tang, the modern American internal arts expert, Tim Cartmell, notes that many teachers in the old days in China suggested that standing (for an average time of 20 minutes) was the most important part of their daily internal arts training.

In the same book, Cartmell also offers the good advice that, in the long run, the length of practice in any given session is somewhat less important than how much quality and attentiveness you can bring to the time that you do stand.

Ideally, I tell my students to aim for a minimum of 15 and a maximum of 30 minutes every session, but if you are very stiff or not very healthy in the beginning, you should gradually increase the total amount of time that you spend in each session. I also believe that you should not exceed that maximum unless you are practicing an equal amount of time of slow form practice.

Along the same lines, I also tell my students that while it is better to do both practices, if they can only find the time or the interest to practice one regularly, they should choose the long, slow form. Standing is good for the spirit and body in moderation, but movement is better for the body in the long run, especially when it is slow, smooth, and rhythmic.

Keeping track of time in a particular session can be tricky. I recommend using an electronic timer to keep track of how long you stand during each posture and gradually increase the amount that you stand in each session. Another way to keep track of how long you stand is to gradually work up to doing a total of 108 slow and deep, fine and even breaths that each take about 10 seconds to complete. Practicing this way will take between 15–20 minutes.

Nourishment

Don't practice on an empty stomach or a full one. With particular regard to food, when your stomach is full, abdominal breathing and turning or twisting the torso, as happens in the long, slow form and certain moving qigong methods, will affect your digestion and you may experience cramps or bloating. Similarly, don't practice with a full bowel or bladder, as "holding it in" while standing will also impede your concentration.

Conversely, don't train if you haven't eaten in some time. It is hard to concentrate if your stomach growls constantly. Have a light and nutritious meal about 30 minutes before training. In traditional terms, fresh air, food, and water are essential ingredients in creating internal energy. If you think of your training as being partly to refine and produce a better quality of acquired qi, it is important to have a healthy diet that contains sufficient and balanced foods while avoiding greasy or sweet things.

Nor is it necessary to abstain from meat or dairy products; it is easy to fall into the trap of thinking that fasting or severely restricting your diet will somehow purify you or make you a better practitioner. Similarly, you don't need to become a vegetarian to benefit from your training in the long term.

I have always found it enlightening that the Chinese experts that I have met quite often are not at all fussy about what they eat and drink and are heavy smokers, whereas the Western experts are often rather pious vegetarians and strict abstainers from addictive substances. But then again, it is often a funny old world, isn't it?

Environment and Clothing

Whether you are in or out of doors, don't train in either an excessively cold or hot place. In particular, avoid standing in the draft of an air conditioning unit when inside, or facing the wind if practicing outside, as your pores will be open and you will be more likely to catch a chill. Similarly, don't continue to train if you are wearing excessively sweaty clothing, as you want to avoid getting chilled from both TCM and Western medical perspectives.

Some authorities have emphasized the importance of wearing long-sleeved clothing made from natural materials (e.g., cotton, linen, raw silk) rather than synthetics, as these can impede qi flow. However, it is important to remember that some modern synthetics "wick" sweat away from the skin more effectively than some natural fibers, which minimizes chilling, especially when training outside. Experts also sometimes suggest that it is important to wear long sleeves and long pants at all times when practicing, as the material helps to keep the *weiqi*—the "protective" aspect of qi—where it belongs, evenly distributed on the surface of the skin instead of leaking away from the arms and legs when the limbs are uncovered.

It's easy to get carried away with rules like this, though, and I think common sense and the weather should dictate your clothing when you train. It has also been my experience that teachers who make the most noise about what to wear and not wear at workshops or in their classes also tend to be those who, by strange coincidence, will gladly sell you special qigong clothing and uniforms in the required materials.

On the other hand, it is important to avoid wearing tight clothing or a belt, as these restrict the easy expansion of the waist and chest for deep breathing purposes. Similarly, women should ensure that a brassiere is not too tight. Aside from the negative affects that overly tight clothing can have on the digestion, the lower and middle dantian in the abdominal and chest areas are considered pumps for energy in traditional terms. This is why it is considered important not to restrict the in-and-out expansion of these areas.

Music

Many traditionalists frown on the use of music as an accompaniment to qigong practice for good reason, as students may learn to rely on such mood-enhancing sounds a little too much or may focus on the music instead of the details of practice. In fact, in my group form classes, I usually get grumbling from at least a few people if I forget to turn on the CD player as they start their training.

However, I think that it's OK to use suitable music to create an atmosphere that is conducive to relaxation, at least in the early months of such training. In the end, though, it is preferable to practice either in a silent environment or amongst more natural sounds when outside.

For experienced students, standing qigong should always be done in a quiet environment, partly because a sudden noise can really upset your qi when going in and out of a sung state. On the other hand, it is also true that it is important to be able to listen to all the subliminal noises in your practice environment without being distracted by them.

It's one of the conundrums of such training that having an "empty" mind does not mean ignoring everything around you or your own thoughts. Rather, it means not being distracted from the task at hand.

Proscriptions to Training

Don't practice if you have a fever or are in the acute phase of an illness. It is OK to substitute sitting for standing qigong if you are injured in the legs or suffer from an acute attack of arthritis. Some methods are almost as effective if done in a modified manner or from a sitting posture (using a bench without a back or armrests, if possible).

Women should stop or moderate their training during menses, or focus on the middle dantian instead of the lower dantian. In fact, some instructors say women should always focus on the area of the sternum or on the soles of their feet as opposed to the lower abdominal area. I suggest that it is important for women of any age to experiment and see what feels right for them.

Don't scratch a sudden itch, as such sensations are often a stage that many practitioners go through. Doing so not only interrupts the postures that you should be holding or doing at the time, but also means that the natural rebalancing of your body is impeded when your hands wander about consciously in this way.

Don't practice when angry, as you are better off doing the slow or fast forms as a way of "letting off steam." If you are interrupted by someone, or the telephone rings, or there is a sudden, loud noise that startles you, avoid losing your temper, as this is particularly bad for the liver in traditional terms. Don't resume practicing immediately unless you have been able to restore your sense of calm.

Do not drink alcohol or take recreational drugs before and after your qigong workout, or engage in sexual activities, strenuous physical activity, or hard-style martial arts immediately after such a workout. Particularly in regards to the latter, there isn't much point in cultivating peace of mind and body and then immediately being tense, aggressive, and harsh while training afterward.

Making Progress

Don't try to adhere to a rigid schedule of progress—such concepts are ridiculous in terms of becoming healthier in physical and emotional terms. Similarly, it is important to avoid confusing the forest with the trees. Symptoms of progress in any aspect of your training can be transitory and should not be the object of obsessive fascination (e.g., "Yesterday, I was 'one with the universe' and it was marvelous. I want it to happen again today.").

Many people practice without dramatic experiences or spiritual revelations, but that doesn't mean that they aren't benefiting from their training in subtle physical and emotional ways over the long term. I have always felt, based on my own experiences and those of the few students I have trained who actually practiced regularly for any length of time, that regular standing qigong really did accelerate the process of maturing as an adult. Leaving intangibles aside, in physical terms it can certainly improve your functional relaxation, posture, and leg strength, if nothing else.

STRANGE EXPERIENCES

Some people train regularly and moderately and never experience any of the following things while doing standing qigong. Others have to endure some or all of them for weeks or months before they pass. By the way, don't worry if you never experience anything dramatic; it doesn't mean that the training isn't working. Everyone is different and many never experience most—or any—of the following phenomena.

Cold and Numbness

In the first few months of regular training it is common to have sensations of excessive cold in the extremities (especially if you are a long-term, heavy smoker or are female) or to feel cold when practicing standing quietly as opposed to moving qigong. Some experts have told me that numbness or tingling in the limbs or hands is a good sign, in that it means that the qi is trying to get through properly in areas where it has been chronically blocked. This tingling can feel like a mild case of when your foot "goes to sleep" or it can feel like the vibrating or buzzing sensation that you get when you place your hand on an electric motor housing.

However, if these sensations continue long after you stop doing your session, or if they become chronic, they might also be the symptoms of disease or nerve damage in the affected limb (or of carpal tunnel syndrome if it is in your wrists). This is particularly likely if you work on a keyboard or with a mouse for hours each day or if you do a lot of qinna (chin-na) training in which your limbs are always being twisted by your partners as part of the process of learning to do joint restraints. In any case, go to a doctor, whether of the Western or Eastern persuasion, if you are at all in doubt about what you are experiencing.

Weight Loss or Gain

As I mentioned earlier, qigong can have a profound affect on your digestive system. It is interesting to note that it will quite often make a skinny person regain an interest in food and gain healthy weight, and a fat person lose weight. (However, my waistline is also evidence that this doesn't happen for everyone.)

Some methods are more effective than others in this realm, and the adjustment is partly due to abdominal breathing massaging the digestive system. It is also partly due to a gradual change in how you approach eating on an emotional level (e.g., if you eat to compensate for depression or being overstressed, such cravings may cease as you become healthier through your training).

It is important to note, though, that standing and moving qigong both can really bring on the "munchies" after a session—especially if the person practicing didn't take my advice to have a light, nutritious meal before training. So be careful that you don't gain weight if you snack after every session and train regularly in this way.

Physical Pain and Discomfort

I'm afraid that some pain and discomfort is normally present in the first few months of training, whether you are doing everything correctly or not. Your body and mind probably won't like standing still, in particular, and will send you signals designed to make you stop. Within reason, you should persist until the pain goes away as your body gradually adjusts to the new demands placed on it. However, you should never ignore pain that is sharp or unexplainable or that persists after a training session has ended.

Of course, you can also be suffering because you are standing with your knees at awkward angles, or tensing up your lower back, or using too much muscle to hold your arms in the required positions. It is important to make sure that your posture and effort is appropriate to your physical health when doing any form of qigong.

As I mentioned before, keeping the eyes at least partially open while doing standing practices is the normal practice. However, if you get into the habit of staring excessively, you can get headaches related to eye strain. You can also get headaches from qi-congestion in the head. These can often be relieved by by massaging the eye sockets, face, and the back of the skull and neck in a firm but gentle downward manner after a training session. (By the way, some qigong experts teach methods of staring at the sun to take in yang energy and, while these may be traditional methods, I certainly don't think that they hold up in modern terms as being safe or desirable. You may well have visions as a result of this, but this has more to do with destroying the retina and over-stimulating the nerves responsible for vision than any esoteric breakthrough.)

Assuming that you don't have allergies, a head cold, or the flu, the most common cause of spontaneous coughing while doing standing training is using too much muscle in the area of the lungs, or trying too hard to control your breathing rate and pattern. Smokers may also find that they have coughing fits when doing even gentle methods of deep breathing.

Finally, even mild physical effort is likely to lead to sweating. There are several schools of thought on this in relation to qigong: Some believe that if you sweat while doing self-healing methods, you are too tense or using too much muscle, i.e., you are doing it wrong; however, many experts interpret sweating as a sign that you are doing the methods properly and that you are releasing stagnant qi and toxins through the pores. The truth probably lies somewhere in between.

For myself, I remember sweating excessively when doing certain methods for the first few months. However, nowadays, I rarely sweat when doing the methods that I practice regularly. By the way, common sense should tell you that if you are training outside on a very hot day, you should sweat, as this is your body's natural response to overheating. A lack of sweat can signal that you are in the dangerous stage of getting heatstroke.

Emotional Pain and Discomfort

On days when you are exceptionally stressed out or mentally fatigued and just can't seem to relax or focus on the breathing while standing, stop and go for a long walk, ride your bike, do a martial form or two, or just do anything physical that interests and stimulates you in a pleasant and moderate way.

Many experts advocate training alone in a quiet and private environment, as you can become very sensitive to outside stimuli, sudden noises, or being touched. Sometimes, you can suddenly jump for no apparent reason, similar to waking up with a jerk while dreaming that you are falling. I have experienced this and seen it happen to others, and it can "disturb and scatter the qi" as the traditionalists would say, so that you feel agitated and upset for quite sometime afterward.

It is only fair to say that some experts maintain that your training should eventually reach the point at which you can continue in a state of composure even if, as the old Chinese saying goes, "Mount Tai should collapse at your feet." But we all have to start somewhere with any kind of training and such calm does not normally come overnight.

In psychological terms, standing can give rise to both moments of great lucidity as well as great pain on an emotional level. Once I started to cry for no apparent reason while having a shower immediately after having done a half-hour of standing qigong. I suddenly realized in a profound way that I no longer wanted to do martial arts just to learn how to hurt people. The magic of that moment eventually faded, but the new attitude stayed with me.

Everyone is different and your experiences during standing qigong will be unique to you. In relation to my own training, a few times I have been practicing my standing qigong and felt as if I was blending with my environment, that I was the breathing process, and that the expansion and contraction that I was experiencing was like the heartbeat of the universe . . . that I was the heartbeat of the universe. I have no idea how long I had been experiencing that when I became aware of it. In becoming conscious of the experience, it disappears.

Being very human, sometimes I crave to have such beautiful experiences again, which cheapens in some ways the value of that day's training. Other times, I focus on being attentive during such training and, before I know it, the session is over and I feel relaxed, refreshed, and ready to take on all the many tasks of a normal day. Some days it is just an ongoing effort and an exercise in self-discipline.

Trembling and Spontaneous Movement

Some experts say that you must experience a probationary period in which you tremble (sometimes violently) for all or part of your standing practice. Others say that you should never consciously induce trembling or shaking as a means of inducing physical relaxation or of encouraging the qi to flow freely through minor energetic blockages.

If you are used to doing meditation or are physically strong as well as relaxed to begin with, you many never experience any significant shaking. Speaking from my own experience, I find that this rarely happens to me anymore when I do my standing and that when it does happens it is usually on days when I was feeling more tense or more tired than usual.

It is also fairly common in standing qigong to get spontaneous movements of the fingers, wrists, arms, head, and torso, so that some practitioners can look as if they are swaying with the breeze or doing slow-motion modern dances even though their feet are not moving. If this happens, it is normally a transitory stage that a practitioner will pass through in a few weeks. It is neither something to be desired nor something to be feared.

Such spontaneous movements, depending on the teacher, are said to be part of the learning curve in standing still meditation, or are sometimes cultivated as something "special." I tend to agree with the first approach and find it hard to avoid feeling that consciously cultivating spontaneous movement (as well as making such an activity an oxymoron) is counterproductive to understanding stillness of mind and body.

Strange Sleep Patterns

In general, the practice of standing and moving qigong will be very beneficial to your sleep patterns as you become more relaxed and stronger internally. Some practitioners find that they need less sleep and function better during the day than when they were getting more hours in bed, but fewer hours of restful sleep.

However, it is important not to do methods that are too stimulating before bedtime (although, depending on the season, your health, and the time of month, you may find even the slow form too energizing for evening practice). As I mentioned before, a common sense approach that I use myself is to practice the most active methods in the morning and the quieter methods in the evening.

Sexual Arousal

Feeling sexually aroused to a greater or lesser degree is a rather common side-effect to qigong training and can be very disturbing to some people. It is important to remember that becoming healthier in general through your training can restore interest in such matters, if they had waned due to chronic stress or ill health. Don't worry or be surprised about transitory feelings of arousal while you train.

Incidentally, I have also met more than one taiji or qigong teacher who claims to teach the secrets of "dual cultivation" of sexual energies (a legitimate though rare and controversial aspect of qigong and some schools of traditional Daoism). Charismatic and unscrupulous teachers sometimes use their interpretation of these sexual practices as a way to entice new sexual partners.

FINAL THOUGHTS

There are hundreds of documented qigong sets in China and probably just as many legitimate variations of each of the main methods. Different instructors will emphasize different things in different ways to suit their physiques, experiences, and their personal preferences—most of the time without changing the value of the exercises. Sometimes, it can be difficult to separate which versions are superior or inferior to others, and it is even harder for a beginner to tell the difference between incompetence and competence.

If you are fortunate enough to have a good instructor, you should learn what he or she teaches as completely as possible before comparing it to what is being offered elsewhere. Without that basic knowledge, it is very difficult to tell the difference between the fraud, the technically competent, and the true expert. The qigong field is not likely to become regulated in any way in the foreseeable future and, while many of those teaching are doing so for the best reasons, there are charlatans (some of whom have been trained as hypnotists or involved in "mind-bending" New-Age systems). This is not an easy issue to resolve, as I'm not sure that strict or all-encompassing certification would be desirable for other reasons. Many legitimate taijiquan and qigong teachers have little or no formal training in Western terms, and some with impressive credentials are, to my mind, the worst of predators.

The methods of standing qigong for health can be marvelous self-healing methods, but they are hardly a quick fix for any chronic, much less acute, disease or injury. It is also essential to understand that lifestyle changes are an inevitable and essential aspect of any such self-healing. It's like getting headaches from refusing to wear glasses when you need them and taking aspirin to kill the pain—at some point, it should start making sense to attack the root cause of your headaches instead of just masking the symptoms.

Any meaningful process of change through standing qigong can only be effectively fueled by a general overhaul in your lifestyle. It is unrealistic to believe that you can continue to smoke, eat the nutritional equivalent of garbage, abuse alcohol or drugs, get too little sleep, endure or provoke abusive relationships, work in an environment that stifles your body and spirit, and somehow counteract that by doing a few minutes of standing qigong everyday.

However, eventually you may awaken to understanding that what you are doing is harming you. But every change—no matter how seemingly small or insignificant—to your lifestyle and your attitudes contributes to this process of maturing and gently accelerates a process that seems to have stopped in many people.

There's a price, though, as many of us think we want to get rid of our bad habits, but then discover that the process of change is frightening and disorienting. Radical change can mean the loss of attitudes or habits that define you as you are. It can also mean the loss of relationships as people react badly or uneasily to how you are changing.

In the end, as the training starts to sink in, and perhaps much to your own surprise, you may find yourself wanting to quit smoking in a way that you may never have experienced before, or you may find that you don't get the same number of colds in winter, or it may seem gross to eat fried or fatty foods, or you may find yourself less stressed by certain things that used to drive you up the wall.

Change is a funny thing, whether you are trying to accomplish it or it just seems to happen over time. We may consciously think we want to improve ourselves or get rid of bad habits and then subconsciously resist doing so, or "grieve" for the fact that we have lost interest in our old ways of behaving. Sadly, it's always easier to make the same mistakes over and over.

However, with proper instruction and diligent long-term practice, standing qigong practice can change the body, emotions, and spirit in a way that can be likened to refining crude ore to produce iron ingots and, eventually, with further skill and effort, turn it into high-grade steel. All three are manifestations of one thing—the lumps dug from the earth—but the final product is both aesthetic and useful in daily life.

To take this analogy a little further, the process of refining not only makes the substance stronger, but more flexible in the same way that a lump of iron ore is relatively inert and useless compared to the sharpness and flexibility of a high-carbon, stainless steel kitchen knife. Again, both are the same substance in essence, but one is the product of time and effort.

In the next chapter, I will discuss the moving aspect of qigong for health—the Yang style long, slow form whose practice can also reinforce the subconscious understanding of the two-person training that is the flip-side to the solo aspect.

Chapter 4
Core Methods:
Moving Qigong and More—
The Long, Slow Yang Sequence

Through standing qigong you have begun exploring how to relax the mind and muscles and deepen and calm the breath while standing quietly in an upright manner that is structurally sound from a physiological point of view. The next step for the Yang stylist should be learning how to move in an efficient taiji-like manner through the mechanism of the long, slow form that is traditionally said to contain 108 postures.

This form is designed to supplement the process of understanding the martial fundamentals of that system, as well as be a self-healing tool for circulating and balancing energy movement throughout the body. The minor self-healing function of the long, slow form is to generate and store internal energy, particularly in the five yin organs: the lungs, kidneys, liver, heart, and spleen.

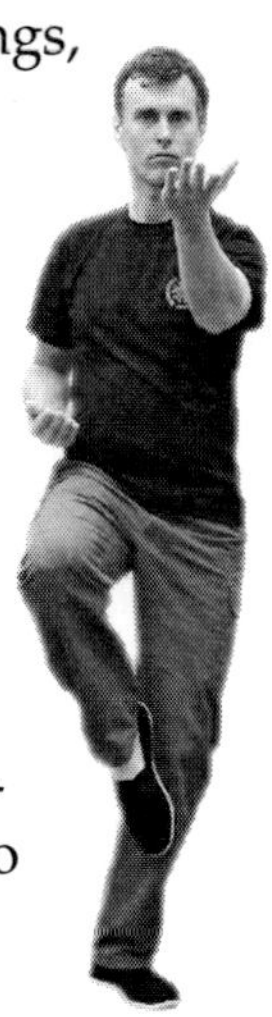

The long, slow form also eventually can be used by the experienced practitioner as a viable form of moving meditation when done slowly and precisely. This is quite unique to the Yang style, as the solo forms in the other family forms of taijiquan are designed to be done vigorously or are relatively short. This makes them less suitable for moving meditation purposes, but perhaps initially superior as martial teaching methods. That may be why the better traditional teachers of the other family styles tend to place a lot of emphasis on standing qigong, as that provides the meditative side of the training that is harder to achieve through their solo forms.

So, in thinking along the line of the famous pairing of yin and yang energies, one can see that both being still, as in standing qigong, and moving, as in the long, slow form, are essential counterpoints to each other in terms of practicing a complete curriculum. This is true no matter what style you study, but particularly in the Yang style. Actually, the first step that most students take down the long road of skill development is to start learning the long, slow form and this was not necessarily the traditional way to learn. I have been told more than once over the years that it was originally more common to train first only in standing qigong and then learn isolated martial postures and combative training methods, practicing them intensely both solo and with a partner before linking them together in the shape of choreographed sets of movements. For example, at a workshop that I attended in the early 1990s, William C.C. Chen reported in a matter-of-fact tone that, as a beginner with the late Cheng Man Ching in Taiwan some 50 years earlier, he had practiced each new posture as he learned them from his teacher a minimum of 1,000 repetitions before going onto the next in Cheng's short form.

Sadly for modern Yang-style taiji, most practitioners nowadays, especially those with no interest in or abilities in the martial arts, ignore the need for standing qigong and have mistaken the forest for the trees. They prefer to learn forms like choreographed dance routines even when they don't understand the martial meanings of the postures that originally made up those same forms.

I must admit that I do not force anyone to do standing qigong in order to qualify to learn anything else in my curriculum. I won't force anyone to learn the martial stuff just to learn the long, slow form. In traditional terms, this probably makes me a bad teacher, but we all have to make compromises in life. I certainly don't always do those things that I know would be good for me, so why should I demand that my students toe the line?

I should add that no one can learn competent interactive skills from a form (despite the nonsense you often hear from modern taiji teachers and practitioners), if that is all they ever study of taiji. The dirty, sweaty, and tedious basics of single and two-person practice are the most important for developing real martial skill—the solo forms less so. In other words, unless they are really only interested in the health side of the system, beginners, for a long time, should only be learning basic practices—including qigong, strengthening, and fighting methods—before they ever learn even the simplest of forms. At the very least, they should study all aspects simultaneously and slowly.

On the other hand, solo forms are a good way to get some regular martial exercise once you have the basic skills and temporarily don't have a partner to train with. In addition, solo and two-person forms are also one way of transmitting the history of a system to the subsequent generations of its students and that certainly has good aspects (e.g., preservation of a competent set of techniques and strategy) and bad (e.g., fossilizing a style so that it no longer continues to develop over the subsequent generations) .

In addition, teachers will often change a posture or two in their main forms to make that sequence more recognizably theirs to knowledgeable observers as well as to put their personal stamp on how they teach what they inherited from their own teacher. Good teachers will keep such changes to a minimum and make sure that the changes are still martially viable and stay within a Yang-style context. Mediocre teachers won't even be aware that they are transmitting something less than desirable. Bad teachers won't care about how much they change what they hand down to their own students.

Of course, for many modern students, going through the motions of a long, slow form can be sufficient for using such practice as a mild exercise as long as they are attentive of the flow of movement and have some sense of doing work in each posture. On the other hand, learning this way will mean that it will be difficult to break any bad habits that you do develop once you subsequently decide to learn about martial applications, as is usually the sequence for learning in a modern Yang-style class.

In the end, perhaps, the greatest stumbling block for the average North American student is the amount of commitment necessary to learn the long, slow form. Many students will become prematurely discouraged with their progress and heave a sigh of frustration when they see a long list of posture names on a piece of paper or a computer screen.

Still, everyone has to start somewhere and it is certainly preferable for students to learn a long form, assuming that they can find a teacher who still teaches it. Sadly, nowadays, many teachers will only teach a variety of modified short forms to suit the limited attention spans of most beginners. Another stumbling block for North American students is the tendency to think that because the main solo form is done slowly, that it must be easy to learn.

Consequently, many who take up taiji as a form of stress relief stop training almost immediately when they find out how demanding of their time and effort a traditional style can be. That's too bad, as the benefits of regular exercise and meditation can eventually help to relieve stress to a significant extent. In addition, research in the United States and in Canada over the last 30 years has shown that doing the long, slow form once provides the same value as walking at a moderate pace for an equivalent amount of time.

However, despite this and its undoubted value as a form of exercise with a variety of benefits, including improved leg strength and circulation as well as better balance and eye-hand coordination, I think that it is wrong to advertise the

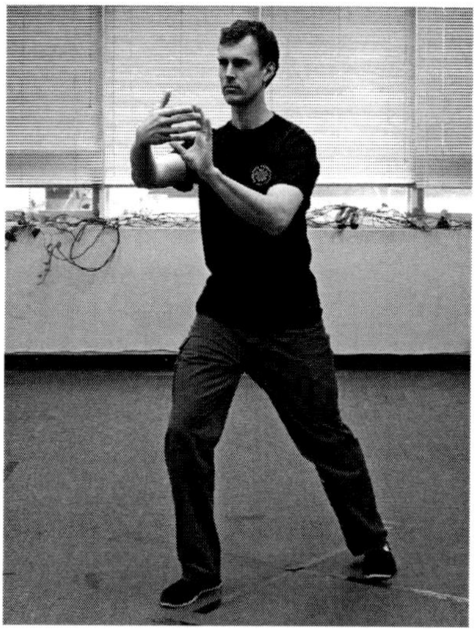

Cal demonstrates peng, which is in many ways one of the key martial and structural applications of whole-body force in any competent Yang style.

long, slow form as a low-impact form of aerobics as I have often heard it described by other teachers.

While the length of the long form makes it a rather daunting undertaking for many beginners, it is important to remember in this context that there are only about 37 distinct postures in such a sequence and that the other 70 or so are repetitions or slight variations of that smaller number. For example, the key posture grasp swallow's tail, which has four (peng or ward-off, lu or rollback, ji or press, and an or push) of the eight key martial actions of the Yang style is repeated many times throughout the form. Most of the time the postures are done in an identical manner.

It would be misleading, though, if I said anything other than admitting that achieving a basic competence in the long, slow form can still take many months to learn at a basic level, even

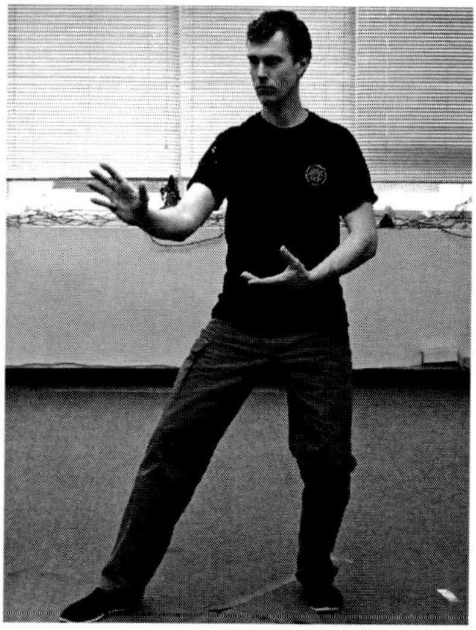

The posture lu or rollback (sometimes called "pull back" in English) that is the follow-up to ward-off in the solo form.

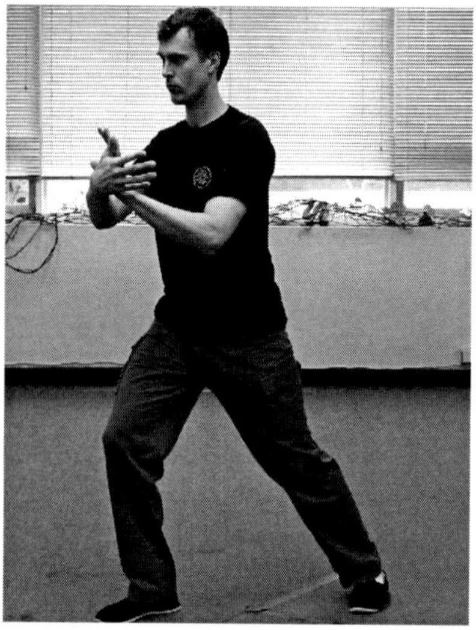

The posture ji or press (sometimes called "squeeze") always follows roll-back in the long, slow form.

if you attend two or three classes per week on a regular basis. And most modern teaching environments are in once-weekly classes held in community centers or local parks. So I must advise you that it is best to develop patience. I also think that it is always preferable to learn the long sequence slowly, say one posture per week.

Especially if studying any or all of the martial side of the system, it is essential to develop an understanding of at least one martial application for every posture. More than once over the years, I have been told or read that a good teacher will teach you one application for each posture and that then you should discover or create 10 more as a way of testing and deepening your understanding of that posture and of the art in general.

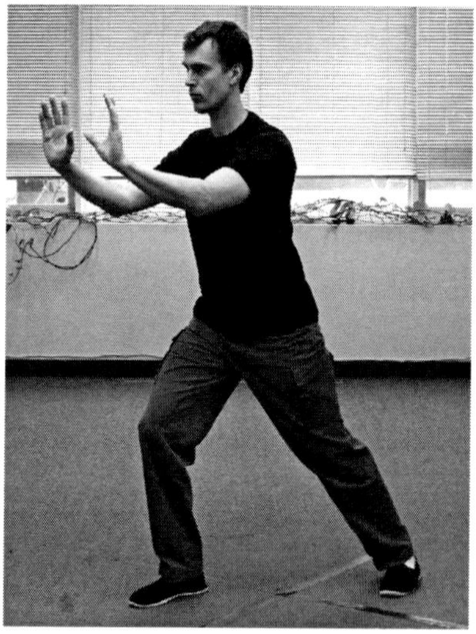

The posture an/push (also known in English as "sit-back to press forward") is the natural follow-up to press/squeeze. This is the last of the four key actions found in the key posture of grasp swallow's tail.

POSTURE AND BODY MECHANICS IN THE SLOW FORM

It is rare to find two long, slow forms that are identical in detail to one another in the various good interpretations of the Yang style. The best follow the same general guidelines of posture and movement and the following descriptions should sound familiar to the majority of experienced practitioners. In addition, many of these will be identical to the requirements for doing standing qigong.

The Head

The practitioner's head must he held as if gently suspended and with the spine feeling "long" but relaxed downward from that point of suspension. Students often tighten the neck muscles excessively in order to keep the head upright and the chin pulled in. Instead, they should imagine a small object resting on top of their heads that is lightly supported. The other way to approach this is to feel as if your head is being pulled upward gently, as if suspended like the strings of a marionette.

One of the saddest sights in modern taiji is to see a roomful of people all practicing the slow form, all slumped in the shoulders with their eyes and heads looking downward vaguely at the floor as they practice. I often tell my students that they shouldn't look for loose coins on the floor when they are training, as I can't afford to leave any lying about! Seriously though, this tendency is sometimes caused by shyness or not wanting to be distracted by those practicing around you, and is sometimes caused because the room is too small for the number of people practicing in it.

Perhaps this is one of the reasons we are frequently told that it is best to train outside, as you are less likely to be forced to look down because of a blank wall looming hypnotically in front of you and close at hand.

Still, no matter what the reasons, you shouldn't look as if you are shambling along or sleepwalking when doing the form. A head that doesn't lift is a sure sign that the practitioner hasn't been taught properly or hasn't listened to a good teacher's corrections. In fact, according to his son, the late, great master, Yang Cheng-fu, made "Straighten the head" his first point in his list of 10 essentials for good taiji (*Yang Style Taijiquan* by Yang Zhenduo, Morning Glory Publishers, Beijing, 1991).

Of course, learning to keep your head where it should be is easier if you have learned the martial training first, as getting hit in the head will go a long way in teaching you how to carry your head properly in functional terms if you persevere in the training. If you are struck in the head or pulled suddenly by the arm, with your head loose and unaligned you are sure to be injured or knocked out—hence the learned or trained response to keep the head centered and upright over the torso in anyone who does a contact sport.

Even though the gaze should be unfocused, it must still have some "attitude" in the sense of looking forward and around and slightly downward, but far into the distance. The gaze should not be lowered even when the practitioner focuses inward to get the feeling of internal movement or fullness. The mind as much as the eye is responsible for maintaining a sense of where you are and where you are going while training in the long, slow form.

However, the eyes are responsible for leading the body in a new direction when a change of direction is necessary. This is a difficult concept to get, as the natural tendency is to turn the head instead of the eyes when changing direction. One of the reasons for not leading a turn excessively with the head is that this encourages the skull to deviate from being both centered and lifted, as if connected to the ceiling or sky.

Conversely, using your eyes properly and not allowing the head to turn means that it can become difficult to turn your head easily, as the muscles that do so tend to stiffen or atrophy to some extent with advancing age and through lack of use. This is why you should supplement your form training with other exercises of simple moving qigong (as found, for example, in the Baduajin training set, that is also often part of the curriculum of a Yang taiji teacher). These exercises train and maintain a fuller range of motion in the neck.

The lips should stay gently closed and the teeth should remain in light contact. The tongue stays raised on the upper palate. While there are different opinions on what type of expression (if any) is appropriate, my own feeling is that a gentle smile is most appropriate for setting the mood and relaxing the many small muscles of the face and jaw. You may find that the type of expression can vary spontaneously depending on the type of form being done (fast versus slow) and your mood. More on this subject later on when I discuss the role of the mind and intention.

Learning to keep the tip of the tongue gently pressed up against the roof of the mouth and held behind the two front teeth is not always an easy habit to develop. (And there are exceptions to this rule in qigong terms. For example, when using a "cleansing breath" by exhaling through the mouth, as is done in some qigong exercises, the tongue will drop temporarily away from the upper palate. Similarly, issuing power by striking while using a "Ha" sound will also mean that the tongue drops temporarily away from the upper palate.) In general, though, while doing the slow form, the tongue stays up and behind the teeth and the mouth remains gently closed. Martial bad habits are often very difficult to overcome and one of these is not keeping your mouth shut and your tongue in place *behind* the teeth and not between them while practicing combat skills with a partner, much less while fighting. Over many years of teaching taiji, I have noticed that a number of otherwise talented practitioners have had difficulty breaking the habit of letting the tip of the tongue protrude or keeping the mouth slack while training. Such habits are more likely to develop when there is little or no contact to the head, as in most modern forms of taijiquan and other martial sports.

It's one thing to constantly verbally remind someone that he or she should pull the tongue in and close the mouth, but some have to be tapped in the jaw once or twice before they realize how painful it can be to ignore the teacher about what seems like a meaningless detail. Oh, and by the way, there's the issue of learning to avoid getting into a scrap that would otherwise never have happened if you had remembered your teacher's good advice to "hold your tongue."

Instructors who have been trained in a traditional manner may also talk about the importance of keeping the tongue lifted and in place in conjunction with lifting the Huiyin (CV #1) acupuncture point between the legs when exhaling. This is done to maintain a more efficient flow of qi through the governing and conceptor vessels that flow up the spine and down the front of and around the torso and head, respectively.

However, there are other very pragmatic reasons to keep the tongue against the roof of the mouth. Particularly if you don't make a conscious effort only to inhale through the nose, deep breathing can dry the mouth out surprisingly quickly, leaving the throat more prone to infection by viruses and bacteria that more easily cross the membranes of the mouth and throat under such conditions.

However, keeping the tongue lifted stimulates the production of saliva, which moistens the membranes and also has properties to defend against such bacterial infection. This flow also stimulates the digestive system, which may also help explain why a very common byproduct of doing slow form and qigong is feeling hungry after you train.

The Torso

The entire spine from the tip of the tailbone to the top of the neck must be held straight but not stiff. However, a common martial misinterpretation of this requirement is to stiffly extend the spine while trying to eliminate the curves that nature intended the spine to have. Gently straightening the back does not mean trying to rid yourself of the S-shaped curves in that structure. These curves are meant to provide suspension so that the structure of the torso is flexible and so that it and the brain are not jarred with every step.

One of the most important rules of taiji practice is han shou, where the first word means "containing something fragile" (i.e., holding it carefully) and the second means "chest." But as "han" can also be interpreted as "swallow" or "inward' in the Chinese language, some practitioners have interpreted this to mean that they must artificially bend or hollow the chest inward. However, a more accurate interpretation of han shou is to empty the chest or to let it do its job of being "empty" in terms of heart and lung function. If those organs are constricted within the ribcage it is impossible for them to work efficiently.

The lower abdomen should be like the chest—relaxed and empty so that movement in that part of the body can be led by the back and the waist. This will make it possible to lead the qi down to the lower dantian. Depending on the style of taijiquan as well as the teaching ability of each instructor, students can gradually develop a strong and supple spine through different exercises.

I think that the idea of forcibly tucking the tailbone and keeping the legs overly bent is not the way to go, but neither is floating and moving completely naturally as we do before learning taijiquan. Perhaps the best way to approach it (in my opinion, anyway) is to remember that the spine and the mind dictate all movement from a whole-body perspective and that sinking or rooting is achieved in part by feeling properly suspended from the top of the back of the head. This is another example of the kinds of logical conundrums that often confront us in the internal arts.

The gentle twisting and turning of the waist should be thought of as the crucial link between the upper and lower halves of the torso. There are conflicting opinions about whether the soft tissues between the hips and the ribcage are major or minor actors in the generation of spinal power, with some experts saying that the trunk must turn as a coordinated unit to support the integrity of the lower back, while others argue equally well that twisting the soft tissues in coordination with the use of the hips and the ribcage is the key to using the spine.

Too much twisting is as counterproductive and health-limiting as not having some torque available to help the action of the hips and legs. Perhaps the best advice I can give you is to find a teacher with a strong and healthy back and take his or her advice to the best of your ability. In the end, the old masters offered a vague but valuable piece of advice: "If the movement is still not correct after the arms and legs have been corrected, then the deficiency is probably in the waist."

To this I would add, tongue-in-cheek, "If you don't use your waist to direct your hands to the task at hand, then the movement is wasted!"

The Arms and Hands

Practitioners, particularly those who are desk-bound in terms of their daily work, tend to have very tense shoulder muscles and a slumped posture. It can be very difficult to get them to achieve an active relaxation of those areas. However, I am not suggesting that you fabricate the feeling by leaning forward, forcing the shoulders forward and down, or sticking the neck out.

The arms tend to be overused in many sports and manual labor activities and underused in the internal arts. The goal is not to move the arms as if there is no range of mobility in the elbows, even if they are moving in coordination with the movement of the waist and the weight, but to eliminate the excessive independent use of the arms. This is achieved by increasing the coordination of the expansion and contraction of the arms with the expansion and contraction of the body as a whole.

As I mentioned before, some of the joints that tend to get ignored in solo form work are the elbows, as practitioners obsess about not moving their arms independently from the waist and spine movements. It is not high-level taiji—although you wouldn't know it from the state of North American Yang style—to move your arms, whether limply or stiffly, as if they were sticking woodenly out of your upper torso. You must expand and contract the arms in coordination with the movement of the legs and spine. This is essential in maintaining a normal range of movement in the joints of the arms, but also to maximize the martial usage of those limbs.

The wrists should remain relaxed throughout all the movements and, while it is desirable for a variety of reasons to understand yin and yang in those joints (particularly for martial purposes), it is even more important to avoid tension, particularly in the palm and fingers. The fingers should be straight but not stiff and separated gently one from the other. The palm should be curved and relatively relaxed in the solo form, but this does not mean "limp." The thumb will be the farthest away from the other fingers and held with some stretch, but the tip of the thumb should be bent slightly inward. Most people will naturally have the tip of the thumb pointing away from the hand when they open it in a normal fashion.

In fact, I will share a little secret with you—when doing the postures of the long, slow form or when training in applications, the fingers will almost never point downward, which will happen easily enough if you have no discernible shape to the fingers and palm.

Maintaining the correct shape, sometimes called the "beautiful lady hand" because of its grace and supple appearance, is another of those apparently minor details that seems meaningless to many practitioners. If your hand is not supple and poised, it is very difficult to learn to hold onto anything strongly without tensing the hand and forearm. If your grip is tense, a more skillful opponent will find it much easier to escape your grasp and manipulate your own balance through the stiffness in your arm.

The Legs and Feet

The hips are crucial to supporting the work of the spine and waist (not to mention the weight of the body) and must be relaxed and balanced. Despite not having a very large range of motion from side-to-side, although each is capable of a wide range of motion in their respective sockets, they act as the leaders of the waist in many ways and must open and close in the same way that the shoulders must open and close in the upper part of the body. Sometimes merely shifting the hips a little will provide the modicum of weight movement necessary to power a posture when there isn't room to move the feet.

The buttocks must follow the spine's direction from the head down to the tip of the tailbone. They shouldn't protrude excessively to the rear unless you are built that way, but at the same time don't obsess about tucking them inward. Doing so is liable to cause tension in the lower back and tipping the tailbone excessively forward, off-center from the natural vertical plane of the spine, doesn't bring any special "powers."

In Chinese martial arts, the term *mingdang* means to close the inner groin and buttocks area. Dang refers to the entire area of the perineum area and lifting this area is often misconstrued as meaning that you must squeeze or forcibly lift the sphincter muscles. This is not a healthy exercise if done to excess and will only improve sexual function (the Kegel maneuver) in certain cases that relate to weak muscles in that area. Rather, you should try to cultivate a general mild muscle contraction that makes you feel as if the ligaments, muscles, and tendons are lightly lifted (as if you are wearing an invisible athletic support that is snug and supportive, but not binding).

During training, the leg joints are worked very hard in that they are always bent more than in normal daily activities (sometimes very bent, depending on the style that you follow). In addition, the arms can rest at times, while your legs must always work while you are on your feet. Relaxation and sound posture (the knee and toes in a relatively vertical alignment is the most easy to understand on paper) help the knees to transmit the weight of the body from the hips to the ankles.

As to weighting while moving through the postures and doing the interactive exercises, there are three major schools of thought on the role of the lower limbs:

- For relative beginners, the weight is never held equally by both legs unless you are doing the preparation/conclusion posture or other means of standing qigong. Once you start to move, the weight is always more on the front leg (e.g., a forward bow stance with the weight distribution being 70 percent on the front leg and 30 percent on the rear leg, with both feet relaxing into the floor at the end of the movement that leads you into that posture).
- Intermediate students learn through example or are told that the weight is momentarily more-or-less completely on one leg—no matter what the stance, forward or back-sitting, in which the weight is obviously on the rear leg with the front foot resting slightly on the ball of the foot or the heel, depending on the posture.

- Real experts often demonstrate, even if they won't talk about it publicly, that eventually being "single weighted" is meaningless in that the seasoned practitioner is completely balanced, stable, and mobile, whether he or not she appears superficially to be double-weighted, perched on one foot, or standing on his or her head.

In essence, the latter expert (and they are very rare indeed) is like a gyroscope in its ability to right itself or like a falling cat adjusting its body to land on its feet. To my mind, this implies many years of experience at standing and moving so that the shifting necessary for easy and balanced movement has become so automatic and subtle that it seems almost magical to those who see it but can't do it in the same way.

I would suspect that every expert who deserves that label moves much in that same way, whether doing Yang-style taiji, another family style of taiji, baguazhang or xingyiquan, or any similar physical activity. As with amateur and professional athletes of any type, the human body can only move in certain ways, and those who learn to move in a connected and efficient manner must, by their human nature, do it in similar ways.

And let's not neglect the poor feet. The ankles must be relaxed and strong to properly lead the feet. Practitioners should allow the arch of each foot to flex in a natural motion—not overly arched or artificially flattened—with each step. It is as much a mistake to lift the arch with tension as it is to try and flatten the foot when stepping. It is also important not to clench the toes when trying to obey the teacher's instruction to grip the earth or floor with your toes. This is as much a mental activity as a physical one.

The Breath

There are general instructions for when to inhale and

exhale while doing the long, slow form, such as: To relax the lower abdomen/dantian, bring your arms down and toward you while you inhale, and to contract the lower abdomen/dantian, extend the arms up and away while exhaling as you finish in any posture. Another commonly used method is to inhale as you kick or lift a foot to move it, and exhale as you finish shifting the weight onto the new leg.

The details of breathing vary for each posture, in part because the timing of the breath will depend partly on the physical timing of the particular posture, as some are longer and have more movements and footwork,while others are relatively short and don't involve any obvious footwork.

The amount of information you get will depend on the depth of knowledge of each individual instructor, as well as his or her preferences on that subject:

- Some teachers will tell their students in great detail when to inhale and when to exhale at any given point in the long form.
- Others will tell their students to focus only on exhaling deeply at the ends of the postures, as this will be in agreement with general martial goals (e.g., exhaling supports striking with a whole body force) and also ensures that the lungs breathe more normally, as you will automatically inhale if you exhale.
- Other teachers will wisely point out that it is better not to pay *any* attention to the breath while doing the slow form, except to ensure that the student is not holding his or her breath from the stress caused by performance anxiety.

In fact, in many ways, as with standing qigong, the long-term goal of breathing while moving through the long form is to do so slowly, evenly, and deeply as you perform the physical actions. Deep breathing in this manner can only support the goal of learning for both the mind and the body, while encouraging the entire torso to feel as if it participates in each breath. Breaking the habit of constricting the chest or taking very shallow breaths is not easy for many modern practitioners.

MOVEMENT

It is sometimes said by well-meaning taiji teachers that the movement of the taiji slow form is as natural as walking. Perhaps if they thought back to how hard most toddlers find it to learn to walk without falling, they would have more sympathy for their poor students lurching stiffly from one posture to another. Some teachers have refined this process by actually encouraging relative beginners to learn the sequence of the form in a rather mechanical and robotic manner before eventually learning to smooth out their performance. This can be a useful way of teaching beginners, although I have also noticed that some students seem to be unable to go beyond moving this way once the habit becomes ingrained.

Of course, flowing smoothly from one posture to another is also problematic for many students, whether or not they are taught that way properly and from their first lesson. The problem with flowing smoothly from one posture to another is that many students get caught up in the pleasure of moving and lose sight of the ends of each posture. The postures start to be one long, slow-motion blur instead of a sequence of smoothly connected postures.

As a writer, the analogy of writing seems to me to be apt: First you learn to recognize and print the letters of the alphabet, then you start to print words, learn punctuation, and make sentences. Increasing sophistication makes it possible for you to learn to write with a script hand so that you no longer have to print in block letters and the letters flow together.

Eventually, most will learn to personalize their handwriting so that it is recognizably their own; but others will still be able to read the sentences easily and understand the meaning. On the other hand, many will never be able to write legibly or comprehensively, and some will get a little carried away with the ornateness of their script so that no one but the writer can read what has been written.

Moving properly while doing form is largely a question of letting your spine, hips, and waist push and pull your hands and feet into position. I'm afraid that I can't be much more helpful than that in terms of explaining it on paper. Doing taiji movement properly is largely a question of being supervised by a competent teacher while you go through all the stages of learning how to connect your spine to your shoulders and hips, and how to connect your shoulders and hips to their respective hands and feet.

But if you are not careful, you'll neglect the key joints in the middle of each limb. In fact, I have met many long-term Yang-style practitioners who have ruined their knees and neglected their elbows so that they lost strength and range of movement in the arms as they focused on the end points of their limbs and obsessed about relaxing the arms and not moving them independently.

Whole body movement is one of the aspects that distinguishes a system like the Yang style from a hard style, in that the emphasis is on unity of movement and what is sometimes called "connectivity." In this way, the movement of the upper and lower limbs are linked sequentially to the movement of the spine, rather than this being a case of, "move the feet first or move the body, then use the arms on their own."

Done properly, to paraphrase one of the written classics, taiji movement should be rooted in the feet and the earth, generated by the legs, directed by the waist and hips, transmitted through the spine, and expressed by the hands. At no time should individual parts be moving on their own. This creates an upward, springy force of the entire body that is often called peng in the Yang style.

A good way of thinking of this in the short term is that the practitioner should endeavor, whether standing still or moving, to be upright, stable, and comfortable.

- When upright, your spine is straight though supple, connected to the earth through your feet, and to the heavens through your head and eyes.
- When stable, your posture and weight is relaxed and centered, whether you are standing still or moving slowly or quickly.
- When comfortable, you feel at ease and you look as if you are relatively effortless in both posture and body mechanics.

However, getting back to the elbows in particular, a good practitioner doesn't move as if he or she has pieces of dead wood stuck in his or her torso, but as if he or she has whips or socks filled with lead shot instead of arms. In other words, the upper limbs are lively and support the work of the torso and leg, rather than taking the lead and acting independently, as is often the case in those who are used to working at a desk or with their brains. Those who chop wood regularly or who do any repetitive physical activity will have an easier time understanding why it is important to use the whole body rather than isolate and overuse any particular part of that body.

Moving Forward

The version of the Yang style that I practice and teach uses what is often called a "weighted turn" or a "twist-step" to move forward. The traditional versions of the Yang style will normally do forward movement this way, as the solo form is designed so that you are almost always moving forward. Other forms of footwork like sidestepping (wave hands) and retreating (repulse like a monkey) are minority activities in terms of footwork. This was a sequence obviously designed by and for martial artists who knew that you couldn't defend yourself unless you were willing to move forward while almost simultaneously defending and counterattacking.

This forward movement is accomplished by sinking deeper into the weighted leg and using the waist to lead the leg to sink metaphorically into the floor through the heel of the lead foot, as that foot turns to the required 45 degree angle by swiveling on the heel as directed by the hip on that side. This is not easy to do and beginners often twist the knee to lead the turning of the body. Leading the turn by twisting the knee is not good for that joint, which is not designed to support repetitive twisting. That joint is primarily a hinge and has limited rotational capabilities. Conversely, some beginners cheat doing the turn properly by simply twisting the affected hip in isolation of the waist movement, neglecting the slight forward and downward weight shift that should motivate the turning of the leg. In my experience, it is harder to teach this way of moving forward and it can be tricky to do on some indoor floor surfaces, depending on the type of footwear that students use. Even if you properly visualize the area below and behind the navel, not your chest, as your physical center of gravity (as if you were somewhat bottom-heavy), it can be difficult to learn to do this, especially if you have not had much recent experience in any form of demanding physical activity or sport.

On the other hand, those with a strong athletic or dance background usually have little trouble with this concept. One suggestion that helps many beginners to understand this way of turning is to try and lift the toes of the foot that you swivel as little as possible and to put the hands on the hips while practicing the footwork. If you are turning to the left, press gently with the right hand on that side of the waist and hip to lead the turning action to the left. As I mentioned, a common error is for the student to just twist the affected hip toward the new direction, rather than let that happen because of the turning of the waist and shoulders—and then wonder why this action feels so uncomfortable.

Whether for turning or general posture, it is important to keep the knees moderately bent throughout the form, aligned with the toes of their respective feet. This is particularly important when in a forward bow stance. It is better to keep the lower leg vertical in relation to the floor than to bend the knees excessively in an attempt to keep your weight low enough. Yang stylists are often told to really bend their knees and use artificially long bow stances, as this is said to train the legs and bring a deep root or stability. Perhaps this is true if your legs are relatively short and you are relatively young and fit, but it doesn't do much for the average long-legged Western practitioner, especially if, as is often the case, the practitioner is not used to regular physical activity.

By contrast, many of the modern versions of the Yang style teach the practitioner to shift his or her weight all the way back onto the rear leg before turning the front foot in anticipation of stepping forward. This imparts a rather peculiar backward and forward rocking action as the student does his or her form. While advancing this way may make it easier to teach beginners, it certainly doesn't do them any favors if they are interested in learning properly. In addition, many of those who practice this method incorrectly and regularly will end up hurting their knees anyway because they've let those joints twist excessively inward while sitting back or moving forward.

From my perspective, the proper way is harder to teach and learn but safer for long-term practice, while the other method is easier to teach and learn in the short term but more likely to lead to knee troubles.

Moving Backward

Retreating is rarely a good idea when fighting, whether on a personal level or as part of a larger tactical force, and the long, slow form does not encourage its practice except as a last resort.

The only time that you really take a backward step is in the posture repulse like a monkey, and that is with a particular set of martial tactics in mind (one aspect of which is pulling your opponent downward with the weight of your body).

Other postures will allow you to shift backward before moving forward again (grasp swallow's tail and snake creeps down, for example) but then again this is done for strategic reasons so that you are not confronting a sudden surge of force from your opponent—imaginary or otherwise—but rather moving with it.

Moving to the Side

There is really only one example of side-stepping in a traditional form and that is wave hands like clouds. You step to the left as a way of practicing avoiding someone rushing through your space (this presupposes that both the practitioner and attacker are right-handed). This is not a way of simply evading superior force, but a way of engaging the attacker to set up a counterattack.

Moving this way is one of the few times that you have your feet parallel to one another and you literally move to the side with bent knees. It is a very good exercise for the legs when done properly, as well as a legitimate martial tactic under certain conditions. Unfortunately, many practitioners either bend their knees excessively when doing this posture, or fall into the posture rather than controlling their weight as it changes from one leg to the other. This is a common error—no matter what the posture being practiced.

Pacing of the Slow Form

One of the hardest aspects of practicing the long, slow form properly is the concept of moving evenly as well as slowly, without losing the distinct shape of each posture that is found within the sequence itself. It is also important to remember that the form is really one long movement and was traditionally compared to the Yangtze, the "long river" in China. Don't think of it as 108 postures as it is usually defined for instructional purposes.

Chopping it up into postures is a way of making each "bite" a size that can be more easily digested by the average student. On the other hand, there is no easy way to teach a group of mixed levels and interests. I should also point out that this way of teaching may well be an adaptation, since taiji started being taught in North America to cater to non-Chinese students. In Asia, it is still more common to learn the form by simply trying to copy what the teacher and more senior students are doing when they practice the form themselves with the group. So each day, a beginner stumbles along as best he or she can with the others and slowly adds a piece to his or her taiji puzzle.

Everyone of all levels practices with a "master" in the park every morning or as often as can be managed. Most of the corrections are done by senior students and are on a fairly rudimentary level. The teacher says very little to the masses during the class and reserves his or her efforts for the fewer senior students after the form or basics class is over. Only in those private or semiprivate classes, where the master teaches a select few, will he or she insist on precision and teach more methodically.

This way of teaching by demonstrating is rarely satisfactory to Western students, possibly because Westerners use less copying and more inquiry in our school systems compared to the Chinese. This is also possibly because Western students expect results immediately and have no patience for gradual improvement using a long-term strategy. It is also true that Westerners talk too much about their training and are prone to discussing—more than doing—in the typical North American training environment.

While it is important to practice this form slowly when you know it well enough to be be able to use it as moving meditation, it is also important to remember that "slowness" is also done to have the time to focus on what you are doing at any given moment in a posture to make your body mechanics and posture more precise. In other words, going exceedingly slowly is only suitable if you are sure that your body mechanics are near-perfect, as it is easier to overwork and thus injure the knees or hips at that pace.

Moving slowly also makes it necessary to pay constant attention to moving precisely and not falling into position as you step forward, backward, and to the side. It is one of the characteristics of movement in taiji that one is never supposed to fall into position on the new foot. The heel of the advancing foot touches lightly and a good practitioner will be able to stop at that point or do what I call "rewind" to return the advancing foot to its previous position. Similarly, the ball of the foot that is retreating first will touch down lightly without the body weight thoughtlessly and automatically falling onto that foot.

This is much easier to write about than to do and going slowly ensures that you are not using momentum to fall into place on the advancing or retreating foot. Even a slightly faster pace makes it much easier to give the illusion that you are moving properly when you are really falling into position.

With time and attentiveness, the form can be done with benefit at a variety of paces and for different purposes (e.g., faster to warm up or practice martial intention and to make sure that the breath isn't being held, or very slow to test connectivity and self-discipline). I tell my students that an average of 30 minutes per session is both practical and desirable once they are no longer beginners. On the other hand, older, sedentary, or overweight students will find it easier to learn the fundamentals of solo form work without straining the knees or lower back if they use a faster pace, especially if it is a smooth pace.

Eventually the long, slow form itself can become moving meditation of the highest order and replace or supplement standing qigong. For example, there are often times when doing slow form that I feel as if time has slowed down in the same way that my physical movements have slowed down, and that an indescribable peace fills me.

However, as I said before, many traditional taiji teachers will insist that form practice is not actually a form of qigong (in the modern sense of that word) as it was meant to be martial training, and that supplementing your taiji training with qigong methods is not necessary. As with all things, it's important to respect the various opinions and then come to your own conclusions as to what best serves your needs.

NONPHYSICAL ASPECTS OF FORM TRAINING

The Mind

The conscious mind has an important role to play in learning the long, slow form and certainly is very "active" when you are beginner. You must struggle to remember where your hands go next and where your foot should be in any particular posture, and which posture comes after that one.

In fact, I often tell my students that relative beginners are doing the slow form on an intermediate level in terms of their use of the mind, even if they stumble through the physical moves because their very newness makes them very attentive of what they are doing. It's easier to pay attention when everything is new and must be digested.

By contrast, the more experienced practitioner can perhaps do the form automatically enough so that he or she doesn't have to pay much conscious attention anymore, and that is just when they tend to start that long "coasting" descent into taiji mediocrity. This level of physical skill allows them to do the form mechanically and daydream through most of it instead of paying attention both to the subtle physical and nonphysical details that they are otherwise now ready to work on at their level—as well as to simply being attentive of the movement itself.

Daydreaming or going into some eyes-closed, pseudo-dream state is not the same thing as the "emptiness" that the old masters told us was the goal of our training for both martial and health purposes. A mind that is calm, clear, but attentive is one that is not easily dismayed by a sudden, fierce attack. A mind that is calm, clear, and empty for 30 minutes or so every day while you practice the solo form is also likely to be that way at least for some of the rest of the day. Modern research has clearly demonstrated in recent years that, from a Western perspective, those who meditate regularly are more likely to be in better physical and emotional health than those who do not. Google meditation and you will see.

For example, I would like to quote from "Buddhist Meditation May Produce Lasting Changes in the Brain" by Jennifer Warner, which was reported on WebMD Medical News, reviewed by Brunilda Nazario, MD, on Wednesday, November 10, 2004: "... [It has been] suggested that meditation may not only produce a calming effect, but researchers found that monks who spent many years in meditation training showed significantly greater brain activity in areas associated with learning and happiness than those who have never practiced meditation."

For those students interested in the martial side of the long, slow form, you can also vary the way in which you mentally do the long, slow form in the sense that sometimes you should visualize that you are using each posture effectively against imaginary attackers, while at other times you pay attention to the movements themselves without obsessing about the details, especially when you make mistakes or lose track of where you are in the form.

Of course, being attentive while being "empty" is a difficult concept to pursue. It is also important to remember that you shouldn't practice all the time while pretending that you are fighting. You want to cultivate calmness and precision, not paranoia.

It is also important to remember that the taiji classics are worth listening to when they say (I'm paraphrasing) that "putting too much emphasis on the breath or on qi itself will only lead to confusion." Those who obsess about how to breathe or how to move the internal energy in and out of specific places in their bodies are often those who end up with very little exercise for their bodies and too much anxiety and stress in their heads.

The Six Harmonies

Practicing the long, slow form properly can lead to a deeper understanding of relaxation as an appropriate ongoing application of force rather than a total lack of muscular effort. I have been told that Yang Zhenduo (another famous son of Yang Cheng-fu) has often said in his workshop tours of North America in recent years that the object of the Yang style is not, as is often said in the Western world, to relax. Rather, the goal of the Yang style is to use relaxation as one of many tools needed to unify the body and mind or, to put it more traditionally, to coordinate the internal with the external for a variety of reasons.

This is a key concept in the use of the body/mind in Yang-style taijiquan (in fact in any competent style of taijiquan and internal martial art) and refers to unifying the three internal coordinations with the three external coordinations to produce the six harmonies.

The three internal pairings refer to the xin (emotional mind or desire for action) being in accord with the yi (intent or the will to act) and, in turn, the yi harmonizing with the qi, which transmits this intent. This finally harmonizes with the li (the actual physical expression of the intent). By contrast, the three external coordinations are the manifestations of the li in that the hands work with and support the feet, the elbows work with and support the knees, and the shoulders work with and support the hips.

A practitioner will normally have the most difficulty initially with the external coordination, as achieving this is complicated by having to move forward and backward, side-to-side as well as up-and-down. Exploring the three dimensions of real-world movement are always difficult when you are learning a new physical activity. For example, it is easier to keep the knees excessively bent or a little too straight instead of using the action of the hips and spine to let your weight rise and fall subtly as you move about. One way to understand this eventually is to pay proper attention to a good role model, so that you copy the example of coordinating the internal with the external.

To put it more simply, the three internal coordinations are about having a clear purpose in each aspect of your practice and of being truly attentive. Some experts would argue that if you have been taught well and are trying to practice well, you will have a constant expression of the six harmonies. If this happens, the movement of your body and spirit will be attractive from a visual perspective, partly because your appearance will be "harmonious."

Strangely enough, this is essential for effective fighting, as you can't defend yourself against a committed or skillful attacker unless your body is balanced, smooth, and harmonious as well as motivated by a unified spirit and intent. I know that this is a difficult concept to get, as common sense might suggest that theatrical gymnastics and expansive movements are better suited to competition routines than fighting, and that real combative skills have to look harsh and simple.

But, to compound the issue, the types of physical skills necessary to do Chinese opera or compete in solo form categories in a martial arts event are the foundation of combative training (i.e., you have to be strong, healthy, and coordinated to defend yourself) and even the simplest and harshest combative action can be done so well that it appears rather magically easy. I don't think that it is an either-or issue.

It is also true that beauty is in the eye of the beholder and you may, perhaps, have to be male to appreciate the beauty of two skillful boxers fighting, or of a master doing form the way it should always look, but so rarely does. In fact, some of the most profound moments of my taiji/martial career have been seeing the occasional example of outstanding skills demonstrated live as with (in the order in which I have seen these, with the most recent at the top):

- Andrea Falk demonstrating split from the xingyiquan style that she studies
- Tim Cartmell doing the Sun style 97-posture taiji form
- Erle Montaigue doing the Yang Lu-Chan form
- Sam Masich doing his Yang family saber form
- William C.C. Chen doing his sword form
- Eric Chew (now deceased) demonstrating the long form of the Wu-style taiji
- Dr. Yang Jwing-ming demonstrating white crane
- Liang Shu-you demonstrating his xingyiquan
- Alan Weiss demonstrating "short power" from the Yang style

These inspirational and beautiful demonstrations of the six harmonies in action have periodically reminded me of why I am still doing taijiquan and the other Chinese forms and methods that I practice after more than three decades of training and two of teaching.

FINAL THOUGHTS

As an example of the many conundrums that confound and amuse those who are involved in taijiquan for any length of time, it is often suggested (as my first main teacher, Allan Weiss, used to tell us in classes) that you should not do the long, slow form immediately after the martial training, as your "animal energies" would be up and it would be difficult to do justice to the form.

On the other hand, my other main teacher, Erle Montaigue, would often say that after he has done the long, slow form with his students, the last thing on earth that he wants to do is practice martial techniques and methods.

So perhaps the answer is to separate the two kinds of training on different days or in different classes, as I have usually done over the years. This, then, creates its own issues. For example, which class does a student skip if he or she is short of time? Conversely, some students choose to avoid the slow form classes altogether and focus on the more interesting (to them) martial stuff, and vice-versa for more gentle souls.

If I had one final bit of advice to offer on learning and practicing the long, slow form, it would be that many modern students seem to have the attitude that the day that they learn the last move of the form is the day that they should automatically retire from classes, start teaching on their own or, at the very least, start learning the next form in the curriculum.

May I tactfully suggest that the day you finish learning how to do the last move of the long set is the day on which you are a qualified beginner. Erle Montaigue has said more than once that you should think of yourself as being past beginner only when you have been doing the entire form on a daily basis for at least one year.

It is essential to gradually (over the years) focus your mental efforts onto the more subtle details that become important once your body can do the basic movements more or less automatically.

When doing this, it is a good idea to concentrate on only one of the subtler aspects during a given session. For example, on one day, concentrate on using the waist properly to move the arms. Another time, pay attention to using the eyes properly, or focus on not falling into the subsequent position, but control your weight properly as you move from posture to posture.

Don't obsess about the details, large or small, or on your progress, so much that you never enjoy your training. If you never enjoy the training or view it only as a necessary chore, you are much less likely to continue to practice over the long term.

With time, your taiji forms should be yours in the same way that those that I practice are mine and Erle's are his. By the way, this also implies that anyone who teaches with any integrity will always remember and teach a basic version of the form in question to beginners so that everyone starts on a level playing field, so to speak.

In this way, if Erle Montaigue was to see one of my past or current senior students practicing a form that I had taught him or her, Erle would be able to say, "That looks like what I taught Mike Babin. Where did you learn it, mate?" He wouldn't scratch his head while watching and have to ask, "What are you practicing?"

Chapter 5
Key Concepts:
Yang-Style Martial Form and Function

Since the opening of China to greater commerce and exchange with the rest of the world in the last two decades, all styles of taijiquan have enjoyed a renewed interest in their martial roots and traditions, both at home and abroad. This is due, in part, to the mainland Chinese government having encouraged a return to traditional martial training as opposed to the watered-down efforts that were politically "correct" during and immediately following their disastrous Cultural Revolution.

This renaissance is also due to the larger numbers of older Chinese teachers, both in China and overseas, who have decided to share their knowledge a little more freely, partly to preserve the art and partly to cash in on the public demand for taiji classes at all levels.

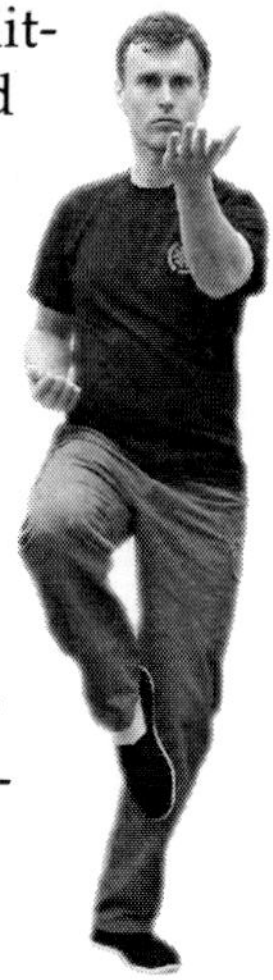

In fact, a cynic might be tempted to add that the rebuilding of the venerable Shaolin and Wudang monasteries by the Communist bureaucrats and the rehabilitation of all the Chinese fighting arts have had as much to do with attracting foreign tourist dollars as they have to do with a return to Buddhist or Daoist piety or a sudden appreciation of the rich martial cultural heritage of China.

In North America, as I said in the first chapter, the adoption of taijiquan by first the hippie generation (rather stiff taiji is being demonstrated in the background of one scene of the infamous 1960s epic, *Easy Rider*) and then the New Age movement led to this discipline—in particular the slow-motion aspects of the Yang style—being seen primarily as a way of relaxing and finding spiritual enlightenment.

In more recent years, many instructors have mixed in qigong and alternative health methods with their teaching of Yang forms and methods. Sometimes this is done to benefit older or unhealthy beginners by making the forms easier to do on a physical level, and sometimes it is done to make the art attractive to those aging middle-class people who have rejected their own cultural and spiritual traditions but find themselves desperate to bring meaning to their lives as their own impending mortality becomes impossible to ignore.

In addition, many schools that claim to teach the martial side of the art only teach push-hands and claim that competence in their interpretation of such exercises will somehow automatically bring self-defense skills. Conversely, other modern schools train with more physical skill and vigor but focus on developing the solo forms as a way of competing to win medals, as well as on the pushing "games" that have been designed to allow the young and the fit to compete in a relatively safe manner.

It is also important to realize that practitioners in the young days of the discipline in turn-of-the-century China normally came to the art with a lifetime of farm and manual work behind them as well as years of experience in the hard styles. In other words, they were already functionally strong and toughened in a way that is alien to most urban dwellers in any culture. Similarly, most would have already known how to fight through long training and bitter experience before their first taiji lesson.

For such as these, the comparative simplicity of taijiquan and its emphasis on sensitivity and yielding (among other attributes) was relevant partly because they already knew what they were doing in terms of the basics of rough-and-tumble. For these seasoned martial artists, taiji was literally a process of refining skills that already existed.

By contrast, the average modern taiji student has never done a serious martial discipline or has no interest whatsoever in getting bruised and sweaty through contact training of any kind, or has bought into the myth of this art being effortless. Many are also coming to class more for the social aspects than because they have any driving interest in the art.

MARTIAL FUNDAMENTALS

The lessons to be learned in structural alignment and what I call functional relaxation (as opposed to limp relaxation) in standing qigong as well as those to be learned from the Yang long, slow form are essential prerequisites to learning taiji martial skills. However, true martial skill on any level comes only from practicing the interactive basics repetitively, sometimes painfully and tediously, with a variety of partners and at a variety of intensities for many months.

By the way, you can get the basic martial skills in about three years of regular group classes. Sophistication will take longer. Perhaps one of the main problems for modern students lies in the North American obsession with progress and change for change's sake. True skill comes from patience, effort, and details being integrated so that your understanding of the forms and methods really is integrated into your physical reflexes.

Having said this, it is also true that eventually practicing only the standing qigong or the slow form after you have already developed a core understanding of the martial skills can let you more easily *maintain* whatever self-defense skills you may have developed without a lot of interactive practice.

Scientific research has established in recent years that even the cells of our muscles have a memory for well-patterned movement. In the same way that we never completely forget how to swim, ski, skate, or bicycle (even those skills may be rusty at first), ingrained fighting skills don't disappear, though they can certainly get rusty from lack of regular use.

However, contrary to what I have heard from a variety of practitioners and instructors over the years, you cannot automatically develop combative skills through form practice alone—this is wishful thinking of the most pathetic sort. And yes, I am repeating myself from earlier chapters, but this is an issue worth repeating.

What Should You Bring to Your Martial Training?

Patience is one of the most useful attributes, as martial skills are not learned quickly, especially if you don't train in them every day. Most modern students don't want to learn so much as they want to feel that they have all the answers—preferably yesterday, although the more patient will settle for tomorrow. This is particularly true for those who come to taiji with previous experience in other martial arts, or in dance or yoga.

Experienced or not, after a few months, If you are fortunate enough to discover that you have some real aptitude for taijiquan, it can then be easy to skip, consciously or subconsciously, the natural progressions of skill learning. I suppose that the occasional person can skip one or even a few steps in the learning curve, but most will benefit from experiencing it fully. Again, patience is the key to long-term progress that "sticks to your ribs."

In many ways, the key to making long-term progress is to practice moderately and regularly. If you train excessively and sporadically, you are much more likely to injure yourself, especially if you're an older beginner.

If you never suffer even minor bruises and injuries, much less sweat or get tired as a result of training, then you're probably not doing enough to make any real progress.

If you get injured frequently or ache all the time and feel exhausted after a group class or your own training, then you are probably overdoing things or training incorrectly.

Another essential attribute is having or developing the physical health and strength to begin taiji or any form of serious martial training. This doesn't imply that you have to be an athlete—although it certainly can't hurt—to train properly and safely. One of the reasons for doing the standing and slow form properly is to build yourself up if you were a sedentary or sick beginner.

You need enough physical strength to safely train in any martial methods that might work in a worst-case scenario. Such training is not necessarily suitable for everyone who might think that they want to do it, especially those with serious health or emotional problems or who are unused to regular physical activity.

While a good teacher will make every attempt to teach you at your own pace and to prioritize the safety of the students training together, you must realize that eventually you will be practicing a variety of martial techniques with your fellows. There is a real risk of accidental injury when you are learning a martial art that might actually bring self-defense skills. You must be ready to put up with the occasional bruise, bump, strain, or sprain.

What Should You Look for in Martial Training?

A good Yang-style learning environment creates the potential to understand body mechanics that rely less on muscle mass and strength and more on leverage, timing, sensitivity, and efficient posture (i.e., "whole body" usage).

Practicing body mechanics that include these things will be the focus of all forms and training methods in any good taiji style, even though the specific techniques and some of the strategies will vary according to stylistic preferences as well as the body type of the individual teacher.

For example, bigger instructors may emphasize "rooting" or the horizontal use of the waist; smaller men may emphasize quick footwork or an upward "springiness" of the lower torso coordinated with that of the legs. A few will be able to utilize either approach as is martially necessary. Doing this properly involves the coordinated use of the waist and weight-shifting as well as the open-close of the body. That type of movement involves the six harmonies discussed in the last chapter as well as "store-release" and "open-close," which are hallmarks in any effective variation of taijiquan.

So if your prospective teacher looks suspiciously like he or she is punching from the shoulder without any body movement or doing a karate-style reverse punch when teaching you how to strike in a supposedly taiji-like manner, you need to consider your other options.

You should also look for a training environment that includes hitting a variety of targets (focus mitts, sandbags, or swinging heavy bags) with some power as opposed to simply practicing "punching the air." It's easy to be smug with the speed of your strikes while doing a fast form or practicing solo, and a far different thing to learn how to hit without hurting your limbs as well as how to absorb or transmit the impact without bouncing off what you hit! It is also much easier to launch a flurry of fast punches when someone else isn't trying to hit you with some skill.

Similarly, beware of any teacher who says or implies that you don't need to learn how to strike properly to defend yourself, as taijiquan is "beyond all that" and relies on sensitivity and esoteric skills that only he or she can teach you. No matter how seductive the thought might be for the timid or those who think too much, you cannot learn to defend yourself—on any level—without mastering the basics and getting a few bruises and boo-boos while doing so.

You should also look for experience with close-quarters physical contact with your training partners. This is the hardest to cultivate in a taijiquan context (good teachers are few and far between), but even the crudest skill at taking a blow or being thrown or knocked down safely will soon teach you many valuable lessons. This also explains why most modern taiji experts with any real self-defense skills usually have a background in wrestling or throwing arts, or have boxed (whether Western or Thai), or have done a lot of fighting when younger.

A lack of experience with any of this kind of martial body contact is the main reason that most modern Yang stylists would have a rough time trying to apply their skills against a real street fighter, or against someone who is really intent on hitting them as opposed to "playing."

For example, I have seen several interpretations of the Yang style two-person application set that were not very satisfying from a martial perspective—like a bad dance without the music. One American instructor I met years ago even assured me with a hint of a condescending sneer that it was wrong to make any kind of contact with your partner while training this way, as you would not be training your qi properly.

Sadly, his attitude is common enough in the taiji world. You should have control in your martial contact when training for the first few years, but you also have to have that contact in some way when you are ready to do so with some skill and safety!

What Should You Avoid in Such Training?

You should be suspicious of an overemphasis on "sticking and yielding," as these essential skills are often taught counterproductively in terms of self-defense skills to make them easier to understand and practice safely in a large group.

It is also wise to question a teacher or style that uses overly complex martial methods that rely on the compliance of a very stiff partner to have any success of application. I have met many supposed experts over the years who are teaching methods that have no hope of working in "the real world," even though they can seem to work in a classroom setting on their own students when that audience is not overly knowledgeable about fighting.

Oh, and avoid any teacher who claims that you can learn to project qi as your main technique for self-defense skills. Common sense seems to go out the window if you judge by the number of schools whose teachers seem to make their students fall over, twitch, and throw themselves by a flick of their master's fingers. Manifestations of this are often called empty force (kong jing), but I would sourly suggest that it should be correctly labeled "empty farce" in a martial context. Most of what I have experienced from different teachers along this line can be explained away as either parlor magic or autosuggestion.

The one or two that I have met who could do things that couldn't be explained also didn't suggest that such skills were anything except aspects of developing listening skills, and that such skills were useless if that was all you could do. The modern internal martial arts (in North America, at least) tend to attract a wide spectrum of students. At one end are those who want exotic answers to life and who want to "play" at the martial arts. At the other end are those who try to make the training something like what it should be, i.e., effort, sweat, and bruises. It's not surprising to me that the former end is the most populous and the most prosperous for those who teach them.

The key to really learning functional taiji-like martial training lies in understanding both the general principals as well as the specific martial training methods and incorporating these on a functional level in terms of self-defense skills. Does this sound easy and effortless?

Actually, I have realized that forms can't teach you anything meaningful by themselves, if you are not experienced enough in the martial basics when you learn them. It took me a long time to really understand this to be true. At the very least, it is essential to learn applications as you learn the solo versions of those applications. One of the reasons that the few real experts that you meet make almost every form that they can do look like magic is the fact that they usually have decades of experience and have learned a variety of systems in their younger days. Most modern teachers—much less the practitioners—of taiji know too many solo forms but have not spent enough time on all the other tedious basics ever to realize their full potential.

Similarly, most modern students don't want to learn how to fight and naturally enough prefer the interpretations of the classics that seem to indicated that "softness" is enough to bring combat skill. Many teachers encourage this attitude for a variety of reasons (e.g., they are more likely to retain students and avoid lawsuits or they don't know better themselves).

It takes a good teacher, patience, aptitude, and a lot of sweat and some pain to learn that softness is best for defense against a skillful and committed attack, if combined with real hardness. By the way, it is impossible really to understand any aspect of practical self-defense unless you understand, in both your body and your head, how to attack as effectively as you defend. There is a reason for an emphasis on yin and yang in taijiquan. Softness by itself is not enough.

There are real martial "secrets" to be discovered along the way over the months and years. These can be found on your body as beads of sweat, in your heart as the courage to persevere in your efforts, and in your head as the wisdom to analyze the theoretical underpinnings of this combative system. I also don't want to sound too hard-nosed and bloodthirsty, as I don't believe in violence or aggression on ethical levels. Many of the moral concepts that have been attributed to taiji in modern times are admirable. What the Chinese used to call wude or "martial virtue"—only using your martial skills for self-protection or to help those in need of such protection—is, regrettably, largely absent from modern martial arts.

If your long-term training only makes you a better fighter and not a better human being, that's sort of sad. If your training doesn't give you the skills that you would need against a committed and experienced attacker, that's also more than a little sad. Without compassion, strength of any kind can easily become intolerance and arrogance, but without strength, fears of one kind or another tend to rule our lives.

Internal Versus External Martial Force

Before discussing any of the general theories and attributes of Yang-style martial training methods, it may help to define the martial force that you are trying to develop. On a mundane level, martial force is an expression of the laws of physics: strength exerted on an object or person, the ability to quickly and efficiently put mass into motion and focus its impact to your best advantage, and to use leverage effectively. On a more subtle level, internal force is also an application of mental intention to maximize the effectiveness of your physical methods while avoiding bad mental habits.

The labels "internal" and "external" in the Chinese martial arts are now so common that their use is unavoidable, but it is doubtful that the originators of the majority of the Chinese styles would have bothered with such distinctions as little as a hundred years ago. This somewhat artificial division became popular around that time as a way of differentiating between the perceived crudeness of the so-called hard styles and their social association with thugs, soldiers, and criminals, and the so-called internal styles and their association with a better social class of practitioners, i.e., those with education or money.

It is true that the styles commonly referred to as "internal" do use common principles, such as avoiding confronting brute force in favor of using the power of the unified structure of the whole body against the weaknesses of an opponent. By contrast, external styles will often condition one part of the body to be used as a primary weapon (e.g., iron palm techniques) and will base their defense on the ability to absorb attacks while attacking directly into oncoming force.

There are also certainly structural and stylistic differences between the various Chinese martial arts. Some are more efficient in terms of structural mechanics and whole-body usage than others, but this is not always because they can be categorized easily as belonging to the internal camp.

I have sometimes compared learning taijiquan to learning any discipline that has both a mental and a physical aspect (dance, playing a musical instrument, woodworking, or any other hands-on trade). In the beginning you crudely copy the movements of whoever you are learning from to the best of your ability. After a few months or years, if you have any ability, you stop copying your mentor to the same extent and start to put yourself fully into whatever you are doing.

Everyone can learn to paint or draw to a certain extent, but few will ever produce a masterpiece. The same is true with an internal martial art, especially as many practitioners are happy to trace their pictures or do paint-by-numbers as opposed to learning all the requisite skills. It is also true that there are few good painters around who offer lessons.

In time, a master does his or her "thing" so well that a casual observer is fooled into believing that the activity is as easy as he or she makes it look—until the student takes that first lesson. The difference between the master and the apprentice also lies in the time spent at the activity in question, the quality of the effort, and the innate ability (or relative lack of such ability) of each.

It is also only fair to add that being a martial apprentice is somewhat different, as the practitioner must not only develop his or her own ability, but must learn a variety of skills that work at canceling out the attempts at mastery by other martial apprentices. Of course, for many practitioners, being internal is an intellectual label that they wrap around their pretentiousness, and not a particular set of physical abilities that can be applied both in solo practice and with others.

In addition, each style of taiji will identify those physical abilities in slightly or greatly different ways. I don't talk about such artificial distinctions as much as I used to for a variety of reasons. In the end, efficient martial ability is efficient martial ability and stylistic distinctions can be irrelevant for real experts. For example, one of the finest demonstrations of whole-body power and movement that I have personally witnessed in the last decade was by a middle-aged traditional Shotokan karate practitioner.

The following are essential points for standing and moving while training solo or with a partner:

- Having a straight spine and maintaining it as the center of any rotation
- Maintaining a coordinated whole body usage
- Shifting your weight through the three dimensions
- Relative relaxation
- Using the mind and breath in coordination with your physical efforts

All of these will eventually become more natural to you and coordinate one with the other, but such skills don't normally come overnight.

GENERAL PRINCIPLES OF MARTIAL YANG-STYLE TAIJI

While it is a bit simplistic to separate the following concepts from the training methods that embody them, it can make them a little easier to understand on paper. Analyzing the theory and mastering the physical training can eventually lead to an understanding that comes as much from long-term experience as it does from intellectual knowledge or physical practice.

We can call the final product maturity on many levels. It is also not too much of a stretch to describe any competent expression of Yang taijiquan as being very much the sum of its individual parts.

WHOLE BODY MOVEMENT

One of the ways to differentiate between any effective internal style, including Yang taiji, from a a functional hard style is the emphasis put on learning to strike and move from the area of the hips and waist (the lower dantian) as well as the spine, as opposed to the localized efforts of the arms and legs that are more often found in the external styles.

It is also important to remember that any efficient sporting or martial usage of the human body will be more similar than dissimilar, as such functionality must follow certain parameters. So perhaps the glut of marketing in recent years, which offers courses, workshops, and instructional videos on topics like Taiji Golfing, Taiji Skiing, Taiji Sailing, etc., may not be as silly as these titles sound—at least in principle.

In this way, for example, a major-league baseball pitcher will throw with a connected whole-body usage that would look "right" to a traditional practitioner of baguazhang, taijiquan, or xingyiquan, even though they would certainly approach it from a different technical perspective.

A competent internal style will also emphasize moving and standing in a symmetrical manner, as it lessens the chance of overworking or stressing one side of the body. The other aspect of symmetry is to make each posture look balanced in terms of what your hands are doing in relation to each other and to the feet and the body weight.

This is not just for meaningless aesthetic reasons (although it does make your performance of the postures look better), as being symmetrical makes whole-body usage more likely in combative terms. So don't stop using or feeling the left hand just because it looks like the right hand is causing all the damage when you practice a particular posture. On the other hand, it makes more sense, especially in terms of making the most of your martial practice sessions, to focus on using your dominant side for interactive training. Human beings, with few exceptions, cannot learn to be ambidextrous.

Of course, this does not mean that you ignore your left side if you are right-handed and vice-versa, only that you focus on whole-body usage that makes the most of your strong side. Any of the elements will work against a variety of attacks against either an open- or closed-side attack if you understand it well enough.

There are three main concerns in creating a whole-body usage in the Yang style: the role of the lower dantian, the role of the spine, and the role of open and close.

Lower Dantian Usage

Although there are actually three areas traditionally called "dantian" in the body, the average taiji player is normally referring to the lower dantian when discussing this part of the body. This "sea of energy" is located approximately four fingers-width below the navel and inside the body.

In taiji practice, you are commonly told to pay attention to that area of the body when breathing or told to sink your mind to it when training. Different teachers see this in different ways:

- A traditionalist will talk about this being the physical center of the body, whose main job is to generate and store refined qi so that you have adequate supplies of it as appropriate for your age. One of the reasons given for breathing like a bellows is so that the flexible tissues of the abdominal area act as an energy pump in the sense of the rhythmic contractions assisting the flow of qi in and out of this key area.
- A pragmatic modern teacher may describe it as a metaphor for being attentive of the body's physical center of gravity as opposed to being literally top-heavy in terms of balance and breathing function.
- A more New Age type of teacher might describe it as being the center of physical desires, which must be balanced with your heart and emotions as well as your head and intellect.
- Certain practitioners may describe it as a literal ball of energy that can be cultivated and taught to move independently within the torso to power certain physical movements or aid in meditation.
- A cynic might call it another form of visualization that distracts students from obsessing about other points of practice while doing taijiquan form or standing qigong.

However you define it, the lower dantian is the functional midpoint of the body. Since one end of all of the largest muscles in the body attach to the pelvis, it truly is the physical and gravitational center for balance and movement. It is the fulcrum between the levers formed by your arms and legs, so to speak.

Since the joints connecting the legs to the torso and this dantian connect the upper and lower halves of the body, it is essential to efficient martial movement in taiji. The efficient use of this area helps to redirect incoming force aimed at the upper half of the body (e.g., a push) down through the feet and transmits the power of the legs and waist upward to the arms and hands (e.g., as when you react to being pushed or struck with the hands).

The Spine

The spine connects the lower dantian to both the arms and the legs for whole-body movement and power generation. Having a straight and connected spine is a difficult concept to do consistently on a physical level, as the concept of "straightness" (zheng) does not actually mean that the spine must be ramrod straight as in exaggerated military postures. Rather, it means being upright, as in not leaning or slumping in any direction as a matter of poor habit. In this way, good posture simply means that the weight of the upper body sits on the spine in the best possible arrangement for support and movement. The aim is to be aligned in a vertical manner as when you are truly so aligned you no longer need to hold yourself together with tension. This marked absence of tension is what allows one to develop efficient balance, speed, and power. The point is to go beyond habitual ways of standing and moving that are counterproductive (e.g., leaning the head to one side, holding one shoulder higher than the other, favoring one leg) and learn an effective and more natural way to use the whole body efficiently.

I have often seen and used the analogy of the spine acting like a whip in the internal martial arts as an aspect of opening and closing, but you do have to be careful in how far you take such analogies. Even with high-level conditioning, the human spine is not intended to be used like a whip, but as a container for the spinal cord as well as a framework for the muscles, tissues, and other bones to connect with each other.

Perhaps a better description would be that the spine is like the mast on a sailing ship in that the structure has some give but is relatively rigid, while the spars, sails, and tackle—your arms and legs—do all the essential work through their flexibility and ease of movement. In fact, I have often seen beginning and intermediate students take the whip metaphor way too literally. The experts who can do it convincingly have practiced such skills properly and probably suffered along the way from their mistakes when practicing incorrectly.

When linking together all the strands of body structure and movement, breathing is integral to the ability to generate power and a full and unrestricted movement of the diaphragm is essential is using breath effectively. In addition, the alignment of the pelvis and its relationship to the alignment of the head forms the foundation of balance and the ability to contract the muscles harmoniously in relation to external resistance (gravity, momentum, and weight).

Sung in the Yang style is often defined in English by modern practitioners as being "relaxed" or "loose" and this is interpreted in physical terms as being like the limpness of an overcooked noodle. I don't think that this is what the founding fathers of taijiquan meant in terms of either the forms or applications training. Erle Montaigue and a few other experts that I have met come as close as you can to appearing to have this sloppy kind of relaxation, but none that I have seen who have functional martial relaxation are actually loosely limp.

This type of relaxation is much closer to the smooth, boneless use an animal—or natural athlete—makes of the body. It is not easy to move this way unless you were born that way. Many students give up prematurely, are content to become floppy, or settle for having relatively loose shoulders and arms, but nothing else.

Sadly, being too loose is even less functional martially than being too stiff if we are talking about defending yourself against someone who has skill or experience in fighting. This should be obvious to anyone who has trained properly in martial terms or has been in a variety of real fights. It is less obvious to the average middle-class, middle-aged recruit to the Yang style, especially those few who want to do push-hands but don't want to sweat, get bruises, or have to touch another student's body.

There's a reason why there are so many more competent hard styles than there are functional internal styles. Speed, strength, and crude skill are easier to accomplish than whole-body usage. For combative purposes, your training should eventually teach you to maintain being upright, stable, and comfortable while simultaneously helping the other person to experience the opposite of those three states of being.

Open and Close

This pairing of opposites (*kai* and *he* in Chinese) can refer to a specific movement of the arms and body, as in the famous posture from Sun-style taiji, or it can also be a common way of describing the use of the whole body in terms of its expansion and contraction. This can be done crudely in the sense of bending the knees to spring up suddenly, or it can be done subtly as in the coordinated and sequential expansion and contraction of the joints in the limbs and spine to create a "springy" power (imagining a Slinky seems appropriate to me in terms of a modern analogy). In the Yang style this kind of force is often called "peng usage."

Open and close is also sometimes related more directly to an inward and outward expansion of the chest or the hip joints to make some expressions of martial force more explosive while also relaxing and strengthening the area of the middle and lower dantian, or the chest and lower torso respectively.

Unfortunately, open and close will only really make sense when you start to do it yourself and understand the martial application as well as the value of doing so for solo form purposes. Even more unfortunately, it is difficult to learn this properly if your instructor can't do it to begin with. As with many subtleties of whole-body usage, it is much easier to talk about open and close than to do it, even crudely.

Breathing: Hen and Ha Training

The use of breathing to increase your strength and focus in lifting is nothing new—ask any weight lifter—and using vocalization to increase your striking power is nothing new, either—watch a professional tennis player.

Let's be pragmatic and use the analogy of pushing a small car: if you don't breathe properly while exerting physical effort (some teachers refer to this as having insufficient "pneumatic pressure" in the core muscles of the torso—particularly in the abdominal area as well as where the psoas muscles connect with the lower back), this results in lacking sufficient muscle power to do the work at hand. As with weightlifting, if you reserve some of the breath after inhaling deeply with a natural pause in the breath cycle, you will have more power whether you are pushing someone or striking them.

In terms of punching and being punched, it is also essential to learn how to use this type of breath automatically, as it saves you from having the wind knocked out of you if you're hit with any power in the front of the torso while exhaling and contracting the abdominal area. Of course, this is complicated because your torso must remain relatively relaxed to avoid causing an impact to topple your structure or affect your balance, which can have serious consequences in a fight. But now we have crossed over from one topic to another.

In traditional terms, the martial use of breathing was referred to as the secret of *hen* and *ha* training. The first word refers to the gentle, rather drawn-out sound you make when inhaling fully to activate the dantian. By contrast, the latter sound occurs when the tongue drops onto the lower palate while the area between the legs (the perineum) lifts gently and, for healing purposes (e.g., a cleansing breath), is done in a drawn-out manner. For martial purposes, the ha sound is sharp, sudden, and triggers an explosive out-rush of air while the abdominal area expands suddenly.

There are at least three sound reasons for training in the use of this form of audible breathing:

- The contractile phase of each breath strengthens the abdominal area and loosens the muscles and connective tissue to provide stability and aid in the absorption of blows to the torso.
- The psychological affect of using a loud "ha" sound at the right time can increase the power of your strikes, as well as your speed, in a significant manner.
- A sudden sound, by itself, can have shock value against your opponent and slow his reactions momentarily, which is often the only opportunity that is needed to "do unto him before he does unto you." Of course, this is not the same thing as routinely yelling as you launch your strike, as the surprise factor is likely exhausted the first time that you do so unless you are fighting a complete amateur.

In traditional terms, the voice (like the eyes) acts as a mediator between your intention (yi) and the qi to lead the hands to the target. When first exposed to this aspect of training, I found it very difficult to get used to the concept of making noise as part of my martial methods—and I am not alone.

In general, adults tend to resist really letting go of their fear of being noisy or embarrassed in public. Consequently, the initial strangled squeaks and grunts tend to provoke laughter more than anything else in a training room. I wonder if the fear of being noticed in public when making noise is in some ways a genetic survival mechanism from the millions of years in which our ancestors wandered about in the wild where silence—while hunting or being hunted—was essential.

Most modern martial arts no longer take such training seriously or only make a perfunctory use of sound to accompany techniques. Real martial use of sound has to lead slightly the physical expression of the "explosion"—not just accompany it. If you make the sound before or after the martial action, you have lost much of its ability to focus your muscles and weight in support of the martial action.

When practicing, ensure that the shouts are both short and sharp and come from deep within the lower torso and not from the upper chest and throat. In the beginning, don't do too many at one time when practicing, as you can get a sore or hoarse throat until you learn to get it right. Eventually, the letting-go process will include being able to "ha" from the very center of the lower dantian—the difference it makes to the speed and power of your movement can be quite spectacular. Like any other aspect of your training, you'll only by able to understand this martial usage by practicing under competent supervision. You'll also need relative privacy, so that you don't give your family or the family pet heart failure, as you must initially practice with some volume.

Eventually the sounds can be as effective without being loud (or even almost inaudible), unless you choose to do so to startle your opponent. As I said, the idea is not to yell or vocalize constantly, as is often done in children's martial arts classes, but to use the sound effectively and selectively. Speaking of which, my youngest son did tae kwon do as a preteen and he loved the large group classes even though I was appalled by the lack of overall martial quality. I remember observing part of one class where the teacher, a talented but young and rather hyper individual, was telling them to yell louder, and louder, and louder until I was sure that my eardrums would pop from the echoing in the community center gymnasium where the classes were held. To top it all off, Mr. Black Belt suddenly shouted, "Louder than that! You can do better! This is a real martial art—it's not quiet and boring like taiji!" So much for professional courtesy!

One last thing on breathing: You will find, in practical terms, that this can only *effectively* be a natural activity that grows out of your training and becomes both automatic and appropriate to your martial activity. In general terms, this means that you will be inhaling to do lifting movements as in pushing someone (to use a popular taiji idiom) "many tens of feet" after first breaking their root, and you will be exhaling with a reverse breath while striking someone in a downward manner, even if the "down" is relatively subtle in terms of its application (as is often the case with the punching in the Yang style).

Perhaps the Chinese philosopher, Lao Tzu, was thinking of hen and ha training when he wrote in the Daoist classic, *Tao Te Ching,* that a baby can scream all day without getting hoarse because it breathes naturally and, by implication, without tension. Anyone who has been around infants and toddlers will know the truth of this.

Being Rooted

Rooting is a foundational skill in Yang-style taiji and refers to that aspect of whole-body usage in which the practitioner has learned to lower his or her center of gravity from the upper body to the area of the abdomen and hips, which is actually the natural fulcrum of the body. Although this should not be achieved by bending the knees more than usual, ongoing correct practice develops very strong legs, particularly the thigh muscles (which are the largest such muscles in the body). A skillful practitioner can become very difficult to topple over as a result of being struck or pushed suddenly.

However, many Yang-style instructors become obsessed with being immovable and such skills can be misleading. They work best with your own peers and are much less useful against an experienced fighter who is mobile and willing to strike you repeatedly in vital areas as soon as you demonstrate how good you are at resisting being pushed from one spot.

Rooting skills also imply that the skillful practitioner has learned to interpret another person's body movements through contact, while creating and maintaining a stable, lower center of gravity in themselves, as when two grapplers test each other in a standup clinch to try and set up a throw, elbow or knee strikes, or uppercuts.

In regard to striking, the more junior student focuses on being grounded when punching and both feet are kept flat on the ground. However, any Yang-style expert that I have seen demonstrate this with any martial effectiveness will move the feet in subtle ways so that the rear foot is raised slightly off the ground or is moving at the moment of impact.

This means that power actually is more effectively delivered from the front leg than from the rear leg even though the latter is initially the key motivating factor to moving forward powerfully. In fact, the majority of Yang styles at least pay lip service to the rear leg being the most important driving factor as it straightens to shift the body weight forward.

This kind of footwork is universal to functional fighting systems in the sense that true rooting actually has very little to do with having your feet planted on the ground. The Yang style tends to approach such matters with the idea that a student will learn to do things somewhat incorrectly for a period of time by always being sunk into both feet, except for the obvious moment that he or she is shifting or stepping, until basic skills have been developed. Thus, using "active" feet and balance are reserved for more experienced students and for applications training.

As is the case in professional boxing, it is almost impossible to get most of your leg strength or body weight behind a straight punch unless you place your weight on the front foot and lift your rear heel in some way near the end of the striking action. Body weight movement and lifting the rear heel is done in every sport that generates body power explosively.

For example, throwing a baseball is perhaps the closest you can come to punching in a noncombative sport. Shifting the body weight and driving the leg are the main means of transferring power from the ground to the striking or throwing hand. Pitching even has the body weight drop, and to this some teachers will add a hip twist for maximum power. Because all human beings must move much the same way when doing so efficiently, there are, in the end, very few secrets left to be discovered.

The Six Directions

This is a traditional way of describing the three-dimensional nature that defines any efficient use of body mass and movement. When you sum it up rather simplistically, these six directions are:

- Up and down: The prime motivation in physical terms for this dimensional pair is the *mingmen* (small of the back) as well as the muscles and tissues below the ribcage. While the arms will obviously move up and down independently to some extent, it is important to learn to mesh this with the action of the muscles, ligaments, and fascia (connective sheathing) in this space between the hip bones and the ribcage. This plays a crucial factor in separating "internal" body mechanics from a more segmented approach as is found in many hard styles.

- To the left and to the right: In simple terms this is related, depending on the style or teacher, to turning the hips and shoulders or the waist area alone from side-to-side as necessary. Again, connecting the appropriate expansive and contractile use of the joints in the arms to this movement is what makes the internal approach different from a more segmented approach. In addition, some experts will say that the shoulders and hips should also have a relatively square relationship, while others will state that the waist must learn to twist and untwist effectively at the end of any posture that involves squaring the hips.
- Forward and back: In simple terms, this relates to shifting the body weight forward and back as well as stepping forward and back. When you add the use of the waist for side-to-side movement as well as the use of *mingmen* for up-and-down movement, you begin to get the kind of physical coordination that is the foundation of any internal art.

It is common for taiji teachers never to have learned about this from their teachers or to assume that their own students will somehow understand eventually by osmosis. In my experience, the first pair I described is the hardest to apply properly, as most teachers—much less their students—will interpret this not as a subtle use of the spine in coordination with changing the angles of the knees as necessary, but more crudely as "Drop your weight there, Babin, bend your knees till it hurts!"

More commonly, as it suits sedentary practitioners, there will be no attempt to use the spine subtly or otherwise and the practitioners will bob up and down while doing solo forms to New Age music.

Of course it is much easier to write this or to read it than to understand what is being described on an experiential level. A simple demonstration by an instructor who can actually do the above is worth 10,000 words that the reader will only understand in his head. Any good style of taijiquan is a "thinking man's martial art" in many ways, but you can only understand it in theory if you don't learn the physical side of it from a skillful practitioner.

By the way, these directions are more about how the body will move in any particular posture or application and not as martially specific as the five directions, which are meant to help a practitioner remember which way to move and how to do so effectively when being attacked.

Applying Jing

Jing is a confusing concept in English, as the meaning can vary depending on how you pronounce it or the context in which it is used. This Chinese character can mean "sperm" or "the vital life-force contained in hormones" or "a skillful physical application of the body/mind," depending on how it is pronounced or drawn slightly differently. So jing could, in different contexts, be a reproductive fluid or it could be an energetic depletion related to an orgasm involving that fluid, or it could be a martial use of force or a physical action like carving a piece of wood into something useful.

Reading any of the taijiquan texts that have been translated into English in recent years will reveal a bewildering number of martial jings that apparently have to be understood by the taiji practitioner.

It is essential to remember that many of these old masters meant their words to be read only by family members or senior students and perhaps by any subsequent senior students later on in the lineage. They were not designed to be instructions for beginners, and such a Chinese teacher would not have imagined—perhaps not even desired—that his words would reach or be understandable to a modern Western audience.

Consequently, when the average modern student reviews these lengthy lists, it is important to consider that the information was for those who already knew how to apply all or most of these skills in a martial context. Those readers also understood how the various jings interacted and supported each other from practical combative experience.

I think it makes better sense for the average modern practitioner to stop obsessing about learning dozens of separate jings and only distinguish a few key ones in his or her practice, as it is impossible to do many of the described jings in isolation. Do I have to remind you that an opponent who is charging you, swinging wildly and powerfully, or launching a surprise attack is not going to give you much time or space to react? Martially, these interrelated skills must be so automatic that they are done by your body and mind in the correct sequence and as the martial situation demands. You cannot think or plan your way out of a real combative situation; you can only react.

The few real experts I have met seem to focus more on teaching their students the basics and encouraging them to understand the martial truth behind "seizing the moment to gain the advantage," as one of the classics suggest. The development of even the core skills requires competent hands-on instruction as well as good training partners with whom you practice in a controlled manner on a regular basis.

Sticking

This is the ability to make contact with the incoming force without being overwhelmed by it. This crucial skill is often lacking in modern taiji practitioners because most teachers will always have their students start the training methods in contact with each other—so that they rarely learn how hard it is to stick to someone safely who starts from farther away and launches a real attack.

Functionally, sticking must usually be applied against a force that is either sharp or changeable or heavy and strong, so if all you can do, or if all you have been taught, is how to touch another person's arms while moving slowly, you are likely in for a rough ride indeed.

Listening

This is the next building block and one of the most elusive, martially. Younger, fitter students tend to substitute speed and power as soon as they make contact or feel threatened by the proximity of their opponent, while older, more intellectual students tend to assume that being able to go through the motions of circling their hands and bodies in a connected manner with a partner is somehow enough to stop a real punch, rather than being just a rather useless choreography.

Remember that listening requires you to be able to survive the initial attack and successfully make contact with the opponent rather than being overwhelmed by that contact. What is comparatively easy to do in a formal exercise in class is much harder to achieve when someone is actually moving in with a spontaneous, much less real, attack. Initially, you must listen with the skin and flesh of the palms and forearms to the other person's arms. Eventually you listen with your whole body and spirit—as well as your ears! In the long run, actual physical contact becomes less and less essential, but this is an elusive skill that comes, if at all, after much practice.

Understanding

This is also easy enough to understand in abstraction, but harder to do with even a cooperative partner, as you need the physical ability to both stick and listen effectively to begin to realize how hard it is to understand another person's balance and intention through physical contact. One of the relevant sayings in the taiji classics is "I know my opponent, but he does not know me."

In other words, once two opponents touch, the one most likely to dominate is the one who has the skill and experience to listen and interpret whether a loss of balance or a badly executed physical technique is a mistake on the other person's part, or a feint done to lure him into compromising his tactical position.

Neutralizing

This means being able to stick, listen, understand, and then deflect or parry a variety of attacks without using excessive tension or muscle in either your arms or your body while still staying within the correct fighting distance and being able to keep from being struck, thrown, or controlled while maintaining your own balance, space, and a calm mind. See, it's easy!

I suppose that in Western martial arts terms this jing relates to the high-level applications deflecting an incoming force rather than resisting or running away from it. By the way, in a pragmatic sense, the potential effectiveness of resisting force with force is certainly better than running away. On the other hand, running away from an incoming force does not work in close quarters, which is why the effective versions of taiji, or any martial art, for that matter, do not pull away from an approaching force. Instead, they avoid or deflect it at the last moment just before doing the last such jing.

Discharge/Explosive

This fajing is usually considered as the end product of having adhered to, listened to, yielded to, and neutralized an attacking force. It is is difficult to learn, especially when you try to copy the skills and body mechanics of the few real experts who are still around, as it is not simply striking suddenly or with a lot of power and speed. On the other hand, being able to fa is relatively useless without the other jings. In other words, you have to have done everything else effectively first to have created the opportunity to fa in a safe manner.

Those of you new to taijiquan as a martial art may wonder what this mysterious skill is like. One way to define it is to say that fajing is a sudden expression of whole body energy focused through a part of the body into a precise target area on another human body. In taiji this is usually transmitted physically through the palm or fist, but a real expert can express it with his or her elbows and shoulders, knees and hips, buttocks or forehead. It is sometimes likened to the power of a really juicy sneeze in which the whole body is involved and it is impossible not to go into a momentary spasm of shaking that involves your entire being.

Again, it is important to remember that striking in this way is an application of the energy of the whole body rather than a specific technique, although each style or teacher will usually have its, his, or her preferences for how it is done and practiced and the part of the body with which it is expressed.

Expressing Yin and Yang

Some of you will have some idea of the importance of yin and yang concepts to Chinese culture and medicine. A simplistic definition would be that these are the two primordial energies of life, energies that are often characterized as being both oppositional and complimentary. Everything is said to have both yin and yang qualities, and it is the interaction between these two forces that creates and maintains the proper balance of qi in human beings, the microcosm and, in all of nature, the macrocosm.

One of the of the goals of any traditional version of Yang taijiquan is to practice the slow form as a means of balancing yin and yang. For example, one can approach this dichotomy in that the stillness training of standing qigong is seen as a yin activity, while movement training through practicing the solo form is seen as a yang activity.

Similarly, any aspect of your taiji training is also said to manifest yin and yang in the movements of the body through the various postures. In this way, the upper half of the body (the yang aspect) will be either more or less active than the lower half of the body (the yin aspect) and the hands and feet will also reflect their constantly changing shape with the fingers and palms spreading or closing grossly or subtly while the wrists also move from yin to yang and vice-versa.

As a more practical martial example of this concept, usually the right moment to counterattack occurs when your partner or an opponent is changing from a yin to a yang state or vice-versa. In this way, you don't start to strike your partner when he is finishing his own attack, as that is when the full weight of the moving body can be brought to bear. Instead, you should start when he begins his withdrawal or starts another tactic (once you have a reasonable certainty that he is not trying to trick you as to his martial intent), as that is when he will be most vulnerable.

If this sounds rather complex, it is, and it is also easy to get bogged down in flowery terminology that detracts rather than adds to your martial abilities.

Intention and the Use of the Eyes

At higher levels, sticking and following is primarily directed by the yi or "intent" and this, combined with the requisite technical skills, are the keys that allow smaller and lighter individuals to develop the potential to defend against and defeat larger, stronger, but less-experienced individuals.

While the normal image of a taiji practitioner is of someone elderly moving slowly with a serene look on his or her face, it is equally true that some of the older Chinese practitioners who I have seen practicing often look more like hawks, in terms of their expression, than monks. In this regard, I remember reading in the small book on Yang-style taiji written by Chen Wei Ming in 1929 (*T'ai Chi Ch'uan Ta Wen,* or, *Questions and Answers on Tai Chi,* translated by Benjamin Pang Jeng Lo and Robert W. Smith, North Atlantic Books, 1985) that it was said by those who saw him practice that Yang Ban Hou would sometimes laugh, cry out, or smile spontaneously while training. I have experienced similar transitory and spontaneous changes of mood myself while doing solo forms, and I have seen it in other modern practitioners as well.

At this point in one's development, the use of intention (yi) is also hard to put into words and tends subjectively to vary with the solo form being done—the long, slow form has a smooth, flowing "feeling"—like being in a river and floating along in a mild current on a warm summer day. The fast Yang-style form can feel quite different and the taiji classics talk of being like a "hawk about to fall on a rabbit." Having seen this in the wild, I can vouch that there is an almost existential quality for the observer at that moment, though it is hardly that way both to the predatory bird and the animal, whose lives depend on the outcome.

In the end, the ultimate goal of conscientious long-term training is to bring a mindless-attentiveness to your form practice. This is easier said than done, and I certainly don't always experience it all the time, even after all these years, during my training. However, the intermediate step before that level is to focus on what had probably previously seemed like insignificant issues that become important as well as possible only once your body can do the gross aspects of the training methods with some precision and less conscious thought.

An important aspect of intention is using the eyes, as all schools of martial arts attach great importance to them—and not just as a mechanism for vision, although it is obviously important to see trouble coming. In form work, the eyes should follow the dominant hand's motion during exercise while also looking in the direction to which one is going.

Common enough mistakes in many modern practitioners include:

- Maintaining a rather artificially haughty and noble expression on the face throughout the form, which is often done by those who compete in modern taiji events, as they want to "look serious" to the judges.
- Closing or half-closing the eyes much of the time as if listening to some inner voice while practicing the forms, which is often a problem for those who interpret their solo form as a way of getting into a trance state of some kind.
- Staring too much at the lead hand as if you couldn't believe that you had digits or, conversely, staring at the floor much of the time. The latter is quite common in beginners, as they are trying to remember what their lower limbs should be doing next in relation to their upper limbs or vice-versa. Unfortunately, while this is understandable in beginners, it tends to become a bad habit, and I have even seen it being done by experts in

demonstrations or on videos while they are piously explaining how important it is to keep the head vertical and the gaze level!

As to the martial aspect of taijiquan, eyes and intention eventually become among the most important aspects of any combative training. If you fail to see the attack with your mind and your eyes before it is too late, then all the fancy moves on earth won't save you. When doing forms or applications you use the eyes peripherally to find movement in your space. If you were "firing" for real as you made contact, the eyes would focus through the target. And as far as I am concerned, using the eyes properly is an aspect of sinking qi to the lower dantian and not a way to do that.

In self-defense terms, it is essential to know where your opponent is, and not just with your eyes or your conscious mind. However, if you stare at your opponent when he is close, then you are less liable to be react instantly. If you use peripheral vision exclusively when you are defending and attacking when you have made contact with an aggressor, then you are also less likely to be able to coordinate your body martially to maximum effect.

An old kung fu expression implies that when your opponent is close, you look at him as if he were far away, as opposed to staring at any one part of his body or at his eyes. An experienced fighter will try to fake you with his shoulders and arms or his eyes at the very least if his attack doesn't immediately succeed.

Timing, Rhythm, and Distance

Developing the ability to remain in controlled contact with your attacker is essential to being able to deliver your counterattacks while neutralizing what the other person is attempting to do to you. This is particularly important at the close range that taijiquan was meant to work within—which is actually the only range that exists in hand-to-hand combat. If an unarmed opponent isn't close enough to get his hands, feet, knees, elbows, forehead, or teeth on you in some way, then he's too far away to be a serious threat.

Unfortunately, most of us are born with limited abilities in terms of timing and distance and it takes most of us considerable exposure to competent basic push-hands and the other training methods, as well as relatively structured contact with our partner's forearms, to learn eventually how to maintain the correct distance between us and our partner at all times, especially once footwork is introduced to the training.

Again, getting back to the issue of the eyes and subconscious mind, you learn to use peripheral vision and an intuitive sense of proximity to monitor constantly where the other person is at any given time. This ability to move with your partner's body movement is an essential step in refining martial "timing." However, such sticking can easily become a liability if both partners allow the exercise to become a mindless choreography and they are content to go through the motions. As I said in a previous section, it is also easy to forget that being able to let go is an essential element of sticking-to.

For example, when doing attack-and-defend training (as opposed to basic push-hands) I have noticed many students are initially obsessed with sticking to my arms with their hands even when it is the least useful thing to do. So, if I seek to distract them by throwing an arm suddenly their way, even though it is not a threat to them (faking an attack), they will quite often do their best to make contact with that limb rather than wait to see if they are in danger from it.

It would be better, to paraphrase another relevant classic, "that if my opponent doesn't move—neither do I," or simply attack me as their defensive measure as advocated in another essential bit of old advice: "If my opponent moves, then I get there first."

Being heavy and relatively relaxed, I am often quite happy to go along for the ride once someone is kind enough to offer me a limb, especially when they circle that limb toward their own heads or torsos in an equally obliging manner. Oh, and the answer isn't to avoid sticking, since if I actually direct my hand toward a target on the head or torso then they must either move their body skillfully out of the way or make contact with the incoming arm or leg.

Certain modern experts, like my friend and mentor Erle Montaigue, have been criticized by their taiji peers for seeming too martial and seeming to discard the time-honored concepts of sensitivity and yielding. However, it seems to me that the methods that these more hard-line taiji martial artists advocate, when done properly, are the purest forms of sticking and yielding, as they depend on timing, balance, sensitivity to movement, and coordination, and not just on reading telegraphed body movements, because your hand or forearm is in contact with the other person's arm.

As I said before, at its highest level, sticking doesn't require physical contact at all, or relying on crude applications of leverage that only work on a cooperative partner. The goal should be to control the opponent's center while dominating his freedom of movement and ability to issue force through his arms. This results in the experienced student having more and more constructive options at any given moment, while his or her opponent has less and less. In some ways, however, the key element in learning how to use these physical skills is to utilize or develop a sense of timing.

Responding instantly and intuitively to a defect in an attack or defense without "stopping" mentally or physically is the key to success. Timing must also be considered from the standpoint of your body's ability to generate and transmit force, as it is relatively useless to stay in contact and adapt to the follow-up techniques if you can't counterstrike effectively.

Any movement achieves maximum effect if the weighted leg powering the hand technique roots strongly into the ground and no blockage caused by tension occurs in any part of the body. The existence of such tension reduces the amount of force that will reach the target. Ideally, this force acts in a wavelike manner, flowing upward from the foot and leg, being directed by the hips, passing through the shoulder, moving down the arm to the hand. Correct timing ensures the unbroken wavelike effect of this force with consequent maximum impact on the target.

While it is true that skill in timing and sensitivity are often dependent on inherent aptitude (expert boxers—whether Chinese or Western—are usually born, not made), it is also true that long-term practice with a variety of partners under supervision can lead even the most obtuse to the "doors of the miraculous," even if it doesn't lead them through those same doors as far as some will get with less effort.

One of the toughest problems in fighting those with some skill is that they will try to limit your options in the same way that you will try to limit theirs. One important aspect of this is that the safest way to defend against their arms is to work the "closed side" (e.g., if he attacks with his right hand, you defend with your left and move to his outside). This is often easier for the smaller, lighter person to do in terms of defensive actions but limits—somewhat—your targets for counterattack, as the aggressor's torso is protected by his arm as well as yours.

Conversely, working the "open side" implies that you defend against his right hand with your left hand and stay in front of your aggressor. This makes it more difficult to avoid being attacked by his left hand, but also implies that you have better targets available to your counterattack. In other words, his torso is relatively open. There are plenty of vulnerable areas to attack when inside on someone, but the problem is that this opportunity works both ways. When fighting on the inside (and sometimes you have no choice), your opponent has just as much access and opportunity to attack your vulnerable areas as you have to attack his.

If you are behind or outside your opponent's arms, the opposite does not hold true. You have access and opportunity to attack his vulnerable areas; he has less access to yours. In addition, you have superior positional advantage to take the opponent down without much struggle, as well as the option to escape if need be. In order to end a real fight, you need to dominate the opponent and, if your opponent is bigger, stronger, or is skilled at fighting, it will often be very difficult to do so in a face-to-face exchange, which is why the bigger and stronger fighter usually wins.

Outside of class time, it always makes sense to assume that the opponent is dangerous (stronger and technically sound) no matter what his or her outward appearance, and that having superior timing, among other skills, may be the only way to survive the encounter.

Folding

A simple definition of the folding in a competent version of the Yang style does little justice to a complex set of abilities. It is just another example of how hard it is to understand the subtleties of physical training unless you have the opportunity to work with someone who can actually do the requisite skills.

In a nutshell, the ability to fold is like pushing on a revolving door in the sense that the leaf of one door moves forward thanks to the pressure of your hand, but if you apply your push too forcefully, another of the doors connected to the central axis is likely to strike your back as a result of your own push.

For those with an interest in history, the medieval European cavalry training apparatus, the quintain, is also an example of folding. The knight on horseback must hit the shield hanging on one end of the free-swinging arm properly with the tip of his lance or duck at the right moment before the other end with a weighted sack swings around from the momentum of the blow he has just delivered, smashing into him from the rear as he tries to ride past.

In traditional taiji terms, folding can be interpreted several ways in stylistic terms and is most easily understood as the ability to move under pressure to change the attacking force without resisting or pulling away from it and continuing to attack. A classic taiji example of this is trying to strike or push your opponent's sternum or face with the right palm as in the posture brush knee. When the target instead blocks my attacking arm from the outside inward at the wrist or forearm, I ride the impact and fold at the elbow on that side to continue my overall momentum toward him as I do a twist-step or weighted turn.

In the two-person training method, da lu, there is another typical expression of folding in which my attempted elbow attack in response to having being pulled down and back is blocked at the last minute and I respond by folding the elbow with that pressure to try to hit with the shoulder on that side. Some skillful practitioners can turn suddenly at extremely close range and strike with the broad scapula in the upper back if the shoulder is first pushed to the appropriate side.

I suppose that, in many ways, folding is just an expression of understanding distance and timing as well as the appropriate use of the intention and eyes—in other words, keeping in contact while following, sticking, neutralizing, and striking, throwing, or controlling (or a combination of all these) until the job is done.

There is no room for faint hearts in such close-range tactics, nor do I think that the old masters understood fighting to be anything but a determined and coordinated application of skills under dangerous and tricky circumstances.

The key factors in any martially useful manifestation of folding involve:

- Being used to rough contact so that you don't automatically tense up when struck or pulled by the arm or, even worse, pull reflexively away. Folding under pressure uses sensitivity and yielding as key aspects—but not the only aspects—of a counterattack.
- Continuing to move forward and through the attacker's attempts to block or counter each move.
- Having the experience and ability to absorb or " borrow" your attacker's contact to avoid getting injured while using some or all of that force to reposition your own attacking limbs.
- Understanding that almost any part of the body can be a tool for counterattacking after folding in the right circumstances. In other words, the whole body is the weapon, not just the obvious tools such as the hands and feet.

I have occasionally met practitioners who could seem to fold anywhere like the snake that apparently was one of the role models for the first versions of taiji back in the days of Zhang San Feng. You know how a snake moves—fast and sinuous, and if you grab the tail, the head whips around to bite you. If you grab the head, you have to be careful that the tail doesn't immediately whip you or that the body doesn't coil around you in a crushing movement.

DEALING WITH PHYSICAL CONTACT

There are many modern Yang-style taiji teachers who will tell you or imply that any contact is too brutal for an art as refined and sensitive as taiji, or that reacting in this way is a sign that your skill levels are not very high. Sadly for those who think that taijiquan is only about softness and an absence of struggle, some form of contact is essential for teaching the basics of combat.

The serious student will eventually have to learn the hard way how to take physical abuse (falling, being hit with some power, being thrown, the feel of being grappled at close quarters) with the minimum of tension or damage. Some taiji schools in Asia train the students to absorb impact through their allowing themselves to be hurled into walls (sometimes padded with old mattresses, sometimes not).

Beware of any teacher who claims to really understand self-defense skills if you have never seen him get struck or thrown (or preferably both). Like so many other aspects of taiji training, learning to be relaxed as you are struck is a complex process that is difficult to master unless your instructor is capable of doing and transmitting the feel of it.

In the martial practice, being used to contact is partly just getting used to having someone "in your face" on a psychological level and partly training your body to take a certain amount of contact. Similarly, taking a punch is not simply a question of tensing up to make a wall out of strong stomach muscles. Doing so can stop some of the pain and impact of a good punch, but it will also more easily disturb your balance and leave you open to a follow-up technique.

Relaxing the torso completely also does not work—in fact, that is the least productive route in martial terms. Even when wearing a chest-protector, a good punch (whether internal or external) hurts like hell and destroys your balance if you try to be totally soft or pull away as the strike hits. The answer lies in "not too much, not too little" muscle usage in the affected area—and more than a little faith.

For beginners, receiving punches must become a conditioned response in which the tissue being hit tenses momentarily on impact and then relaxes once the power is removed. Learning to do this is difficult but not impossible and it's not just a question of autosuggestion so that you ignore the pain. Once you learn how to receive a basic punch (i.e., the power comes from the arm rather than the weight of the attacker or the attacker doesn't step through his target properly), the impact to the torso won't hurt and doesn't affect your balance. You also don't get bruising or internal damage afterward, unless you are hit particularly well on a particularly vulnerable point.

A whole-body punch from someone who steps through the target is much harder to deal with, but that is why the seasoned practitioner learns to turn or deflect the impact through moving his body properly to help deflect or erode more committed strikes.

Assuming that your taiji teacher can't or won't teach you such contact skills, the easiest way to learn these days is to take up Western boxing. Any good boxer learns to take pain and impact without getting internal injuries as a byproduct of the training. There are lots of ex-boxers around and you rarely hear of them dying or becoming invalids because of internal injuries to the torso.

It's also true that Western boxing on a professional level is liable to lead to long-term brain damage in even the finest fighter, so that should be a consideration as well. It's the blows to the head that are problematic and usually cause long-term disabilities.

Those nights that I have "a bit o' the devil in me," I'll let one of my newer students put on the boxing gloves and try to hit me in the lower torso before I can touch him. This is both an excellent training method and a bit of a dirty trick, as when you stand close enough (i.e., within fighting range), it is very difficult for your partner to hit you before you touch them if you are relaxed enough not to telegraph your movements.

So the poor student stands there and I'm touching him relatively slowly and gently on the shoulder or face while he fires too late and, when he does hit me with some power, he knocks himself over because he's not used to hitting someone who is used to being hit. The punches bounce or slide off because of the student's relative stiffness, or the student wonders at how someone he or she has just punched vigorously can stand there and smile while being hit!

Still, having learned to take a punch, I know how hard it is to remain relaxed while some stranger is smiling or trying to look like a hard-ass while winding-up! As I mentioned, a traditionalist might argue that it is also important to circulate and pack the qi into the area being struck. Learning to do the latter involves learning and practicing iron shirt qigong—many styles having once been available and having faith combined with affective physical techniques.

Iron shirt or golden bell conditioning methods are all versions of the same traditional training, whose goal was to teach the fighter to deal with blows to certain parts of the body.[1] In traditional kung fu and in some taiji schools, learning to hit yourself is often a precursor to learning to take contact from someone else. These methods can be as simple as shifting the weight from one leg to the other and swinging the arms from front to back through the rotation of the spine. The impact of the closed hands on the torso is said to toughen the skin and stimulate the flow of qi to the surface.

Variations of this are done lightly in qigong for health to stimulate the kidneys and "protective energy" or weiqi (e.g., hawker beats his drum). More vigorous versions are done with greater impact and speed and use particular ways of breathing each time a hand makes contact with the torso. Other methods involve hitting the limbs and torso rhythmically or having someone else do this with gradually increasing force—either with a hand or a variety of objects (e.g., sticks of various diameter, or pebbles in a leather bag).

By the way, such skills are relatively useless unless those doing so also learn how to take the fight effectively to the attacker. While it is certainly better to give than to receive (to paraphrase from an excellent old Christian "classic"), it is also true that even the best fighter may get hit. Being used to that contact is what makes him or her capable in the first place.

Such training was not normally considered suitable for soldiers because of the need to train large numbers of recruits to go to war within a few weeks, not after many months of training. Instead, the training methods I am aware of in the taiji universe were gradual and incremental (e.g., striking yourself increasingly harder as part of this kind of qigong training, or doing two-person conditioning methods, or hitting the body with a leather bag to which you would add one pebble per day over a course of many months) and aimed as much at stimulating the qi and internal organs as creating unarmed fighting skills.

It is also important to note that many modern teachers deny the existence of such training in their traditions in a misguided attempt to protect their "secrets." Others will say that such specific training is unnecessary because the practitioner's body will get used to being hit simply through the regular training. This is certainly true enough for those with the will to learn, but I doubt that the average modern taiji student has much hope of learning to take a punch of any kind to the torso without training specifically to learn such skills.

On the other hand, I no longer think that it is essential to do specific iron shirt qigong methods, but I also don't regret the time that I spent practicing the traditional qigong sets that I did learn years ago. In modern terms, a younger, fitter person is better off learning wrestling or judo or any contact sport in some ways, as many of the traditional methods you come across are rather extreme and pose a risk for the naive Westerner being exploited in physical, emotional, or financial terms by an unscrupulous teacher.

However you approach being a human "heavy bag," understanding how to do reverse abdominal breathing is essential. Similarly, doing regular standing qigong is essential both for good health and having a normal amount of weiqi, which is the protective aspect of internal energy. Pragmatically, it is impossible to know if the weiqi really does flow to the surface of the skin when you are struck, but if you can visualize this as happening, it helps in the early stages of your training.

I have also had some success in teaching this by using a more modern analogy. I tell the student to imagine that the push of the bare hand or the blow from a gloved fist on their torso activates a science-fiction type of force-shield and that this absorbs the attacker's force and uses it to charge your own follow-up action. What is excess to its requirements is automatically blown back or rebounded to the attacker.

When learning to receive punches to the torso, it is essential that you be able to feel how the instructor does this if you are to hope to copy this torso application of peng. As in all aspects of internal training, you need competent instruction, faith in the method you learn, the willingness or need to learn it, a good training partner you can trust, and perseverance.

As to the techniques, these are best learned from someone who can do them. Expect some pain and bruising in the beginning. This is where the old Chinese kung fu expression, "Not to beat is to cheat the student," becomes relevant, since it is by feeling how the teacher expresses his power that a good student will learn to do the same thing with others.

Although a particularly talented student might come to understand these things through his or her own investigations, this process of energy and tactile transmission is more direct and sure and is a most important part of the traditional student and teacher relationship. I think of it as "inoculating" my senior students with the ability to strike properly by doing it to them. Other teachers refer to it in other ways.

While I have taught a variety of exercises, including some that involve receiving and returning a medicine ball as well as real punches to the torso with a both a boxing gloved hand and a bare-hand punch, this is well beyond learning from a written description. The old masters were correct in repeating endlessly that there is no substitute for personal instruction.

The following training is the only one that I teach that is relatively safe to experiment with on your own if you are curious about this concept of how contact of any kind changes the parameters of your taiji training.

RECEIVING AND RETURNING

This method is the result of my experimentation, although it is based on methods used by a variety of internal experts whom I have met or studied with over the years.

A pair of students stand with their feet shoulder-width apart, one foot slightly in front of the other, while facing each other. One student has his or her left foot slightly forward and the partner does the reverse stance. They should be close enough to each other so that their elbows remain comfortably bent even when the arms are extended.

One person (the "sender") puts his open palm on the other person's lower torso and pushes slowly and firmly into the other person (the "receiver"), who also has his or her hand on the sender's lower torso. The sender should have a balanced approach to how much force he or she uses. Too much strength and you'll push the person over, if you're bigger. If you're smaller, your arms will soon get tired, especially if your partner resists skillfully.

Initially using the open hand as well as relatively slow and gentle pushing is less threatening (or painful) than punching each other and lets you learn to "listen" with both your palm and your torso where the other person's hand is in contact.

Try to avoid tensing when receiving a push and while trying to return it with the gentle inflation of the abdomen, the twisting of the spine, and a minimum of physical movement or effort in the affected arm.

At first, practice only with a partner who is roughly your height and weight or who has a great deal of control. Eventually, height, weight, and arm reach become less deciding factors, although the shorter person should always decide the range between two players by reaching forward so that he or she can easily touch the taller person's torso with a palm.

The main rule is for the sender to keep his or her balance, not use too much muscle, and not move his or her feet while pushing the receiver into moving his or her feet. Use a timer to create short rounds (two to three minutes) and switch partners when the beeper sounds. Remember to push smoothly and not to "strike" in any way (i.e., make sudden movements) and to practice on both sides. If your right hand is on your partner, then your right foot should be slightly forward (i.e., a "natural" stance). Don't use a reverse stance, as this makes it easier to push by using the legs in a subtle manner.

Take turns being the sender and remember that the idea is to move the arms and legs as little as possible while receiving the push and trying to help the other person fall over if his or her push is stiffer than your "returning." Oh, and there are many ways to cheat:

- Leaning subtly or not-so-subtly into your partner, particularly if you are taller than him or her.
- Over-bending the knees and then springing with too much muscle and speed instead of also using the spine when returning the push.
- Resisting the push and then just using upper body force to try and get the other person to move.

Dealing with a downward push is the easiest for anyone with rooting and relaxing skill. Dealing with a straight-ahead energy is harder and deflecting an upward push is the hardest of all.

If both partners have roughly the same level of skill and are roughly the same size, the exercise can easily turn into a stalemate in which neither seems, to a casual observer, to be doing much. When this happens you need a different partner or you need to move onto the "advanced" versions of this exercise, but those can't and shouldn't be learned from a book.

THE FIVE PILLARS OF YANG-STYLE MARTIAL TRAINING

I have already briefly described the curriculum that I am using in my martial Yang taiji classes in an earlier chapter, but few teachers will agree on what constitutes a complete approach to training in this style. Most modern schools of the Yang style will teach only the slow form and some qigong exercises. A few will teach different kinds of push-hands and call that their martial training. Some will say or imply that that is all the training that is needed beside the long, slow form to somehow bring superior martial skills.

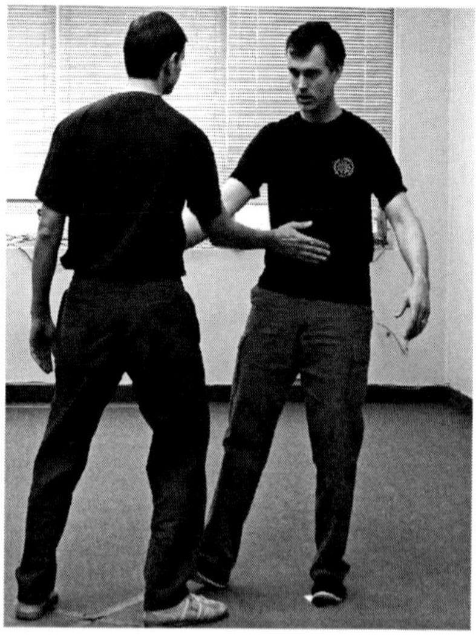

Cal (facing the camera) has pushed into Alan's torso and been bounced back by Alan's skillful returning of the energy of the push

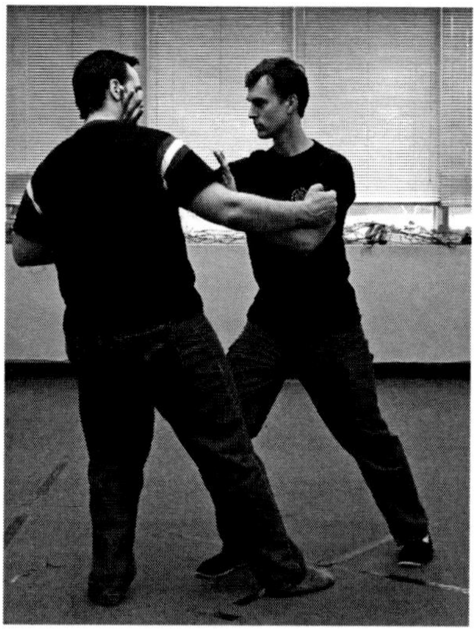

Grasp swallow's tail applications: peng. Mike throws a punch and Cal has deflected with the left hand while moving forward so that his right hand strikes the neck or side of the face

The majority of modern taijiquan practitioners should watch a number of mixed martial arts (MMA) fights either live or on television to get some understanding of why most combative training in any taijiquan style is pretty tame and more than a little lame. Of course, most taiji practitioners who watch such extreme sports will rightly express their disgust over the brutal nature of such events but then go back to doing what they have always done in push-hands training and continue to think they're superior to the bruised and bloodied athletes they have seen contend in a ring or cage.

For all my shortcomings as a taiji practitioner, martial artist, and teacher, I

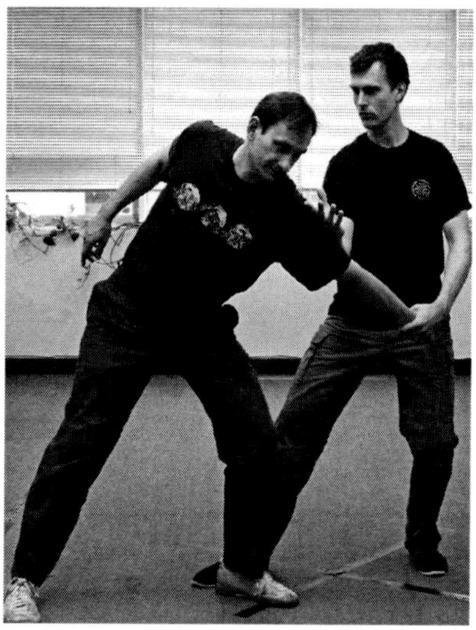

Grasp swallow's tail applications: pullback. Cal shifts backward and applies a downward arm bar to Alan. This can harm the elbow as well as jerk Alan into the floor if he responds stiffly. Controlling the wrist first is essential to make this kind of control possible, as is the positioning of Cal's right hand on Alan's elbow.

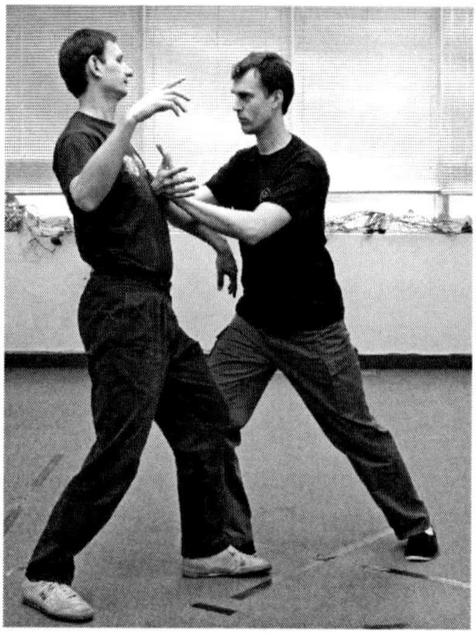

Grasp swallow's tail applications: press. This is a natural follow-up to the previous posture of pullback, especially if Alan has resisted being pulled downward and Cal takes advantage of this to move forward suddenly. This action can be used as a strike or a push.

have learned how to get hit and how to deal with spontaneous attacks within the limited context of a friendly training environment, which puts me in the position of at least knowing what I can't do! Most of my colleagues, much less their students, should open their eyes a little when it comes to understanding what makes someone capable of defending themselves in any martial context.

Keeping this in mind, I agree with the minority of modern experts who argue that push-hands and related exercises should be learned after having gained some skill at posture applications and the long two-person set. At a minimum, I also feel that it is essential that the five following training methods be present in any modern system

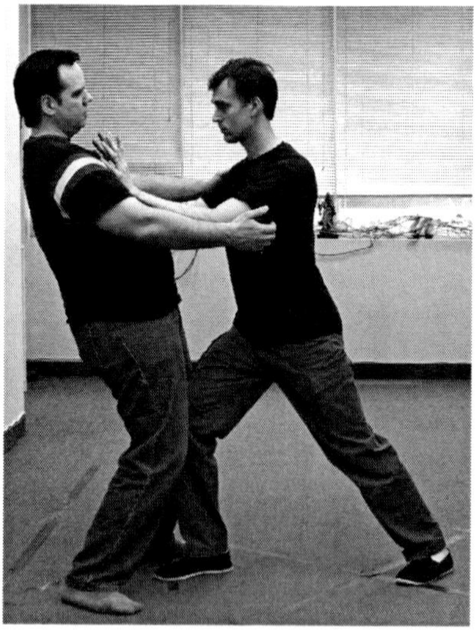

Grasp swallow's tail applications: push. This can be used as a preemptive strike at close range and Cal's lead foot can be trapping Mike's foot to make it more likely that Mike will stumble or fall because of the impact.

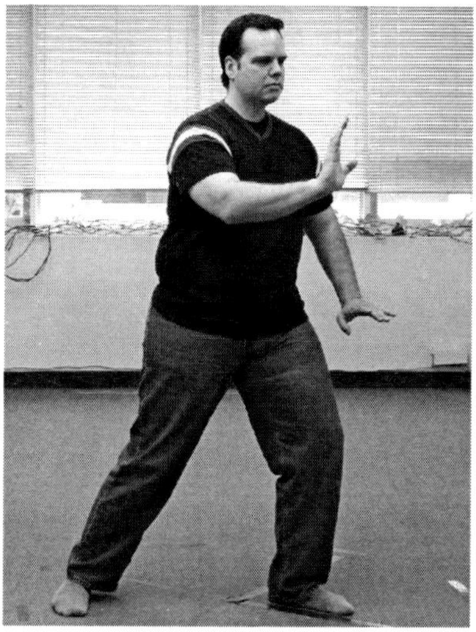

Brush knee solo.

that hopes to provide even a pale reflection of what the Yang style can be as a serious martial system.

One: Posture Applications

In the chapter on the solo practice of the slow form, I mentioned how important it is to develop some concept of what each posture means. However, to learn any such posture on a meaningful martial level, you will have to isolate and practice individual techniques many times with a variety of training partners and at a variety of intensities as your understanding and skills develop.

Such interaction, even when done slowly and carefully, complicates and changes your feel for the mechanics of each posture. Now you really begin to learn where your hands and feet should be at any one time, how to get them there using taiji principles, and how to relax "under pressure." As in all aspects of taiji, it is much easier to talk about practicing applications safely and effectively than it is to do them.

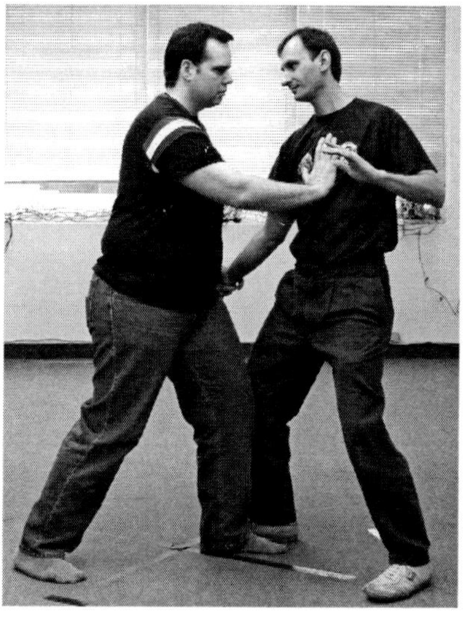

Brush knee as an application.

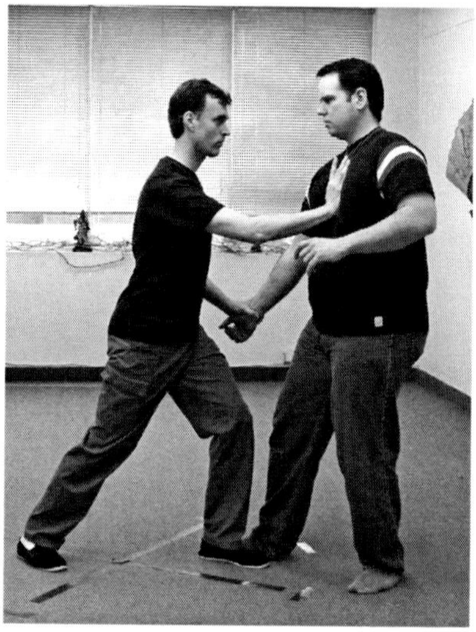

Cal has hit or tried to hit Mike using brush knee.

Another good example of a frequently repeated posture in the the Yang style that allows for rapid-fire striking is chop with fist. In most variations that I have seen, it looks as if you have stepped once into a right leg bow stance, but this seemingly simple transition includes a potential elbow strike followed by a right backfist and a left palm strike. These can be delivered rapid fire if the attack collapses, or theycan be used to deflect and neutralize several incoming follow-up strikes as you counterattack.

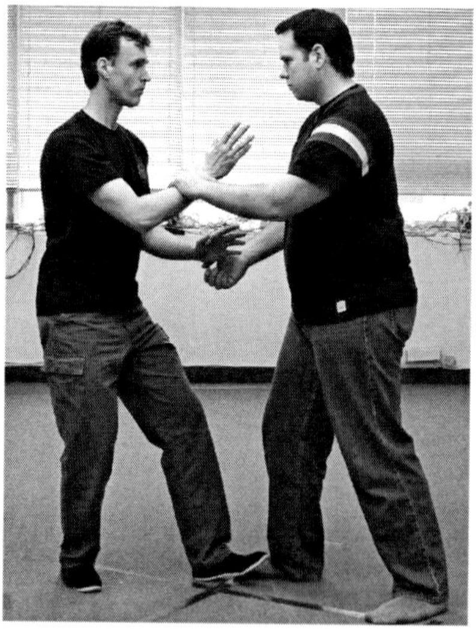

There is a good martial reason that chop with fist and what I call its big brother, step up to deflect parry and punch, are repeated so many times in traditional versions of the long, slow Yang form, as the latter posture adds a low kick and following-up if the attacker backpedals and you must continue to "stick to and not let go."

Mike rides the impact and grabs Cal's hand to jam it into him.

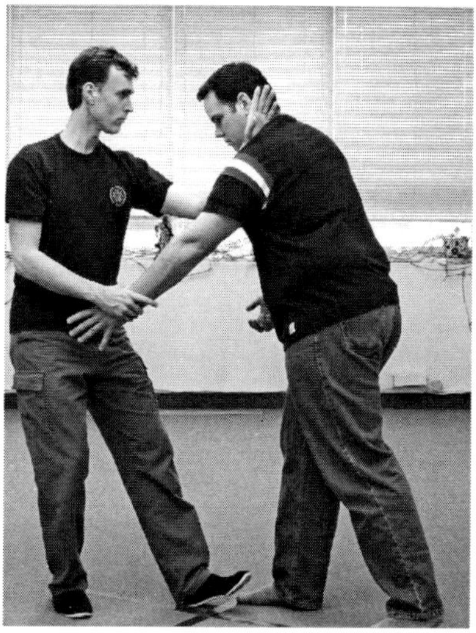

Cal rides the force he is given and shifts back to apply play the lute as a strike to the neck.

In the long, slow form, play the lute appears with brush knee, as the former is a natural follow-up if an attacker pushes or steps toward you after having stopped your palm strike with the latter. You allow your body to go back in response to that forward pressure to lock or momentarily control the pushing arm and kick with the left foot as it empties.

Play the lute can also be used to a deflect a high punch while counterstriking to the neck and or face. The same energy is manifested in da lu and uses more footwork to move out of the way of a shoulder or elbow strike while controlling the attacker's lead arm and slapping the ear or neck.

When done properly (the way I learned it, anyway), there is a twisting energy to either application that suits the analogy of running into a clothesline at neck-height. In the other modern versions that I have seen, there is usually only one major direction

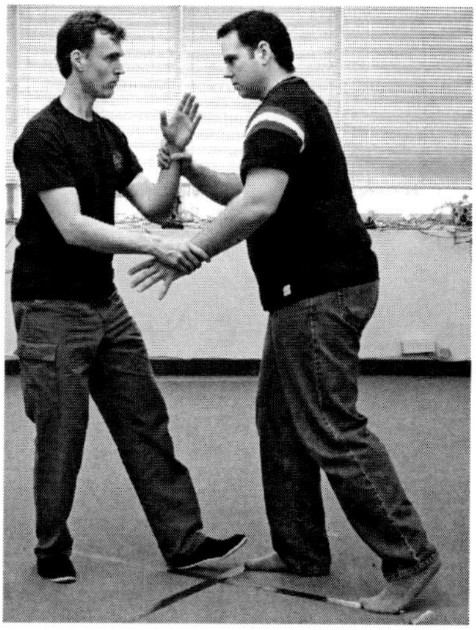

Mike again grabs and counters the hand threatening his neck.

Cal reacts before Mike can strike him and upsets his opponent's balance by applying the transitional hold the ball movement within brush knee.

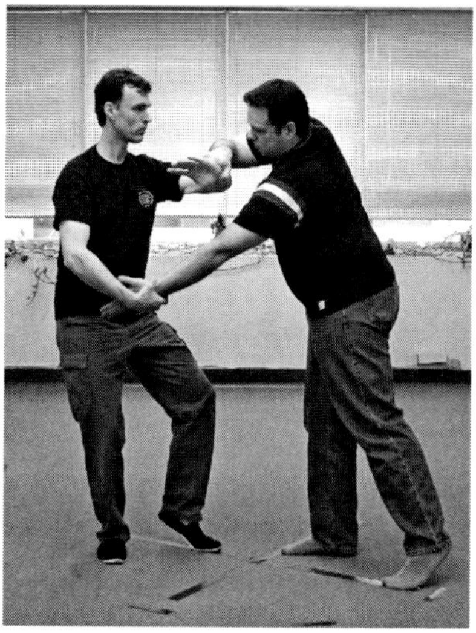

used—and usually that is an energy that moves horizontally from out to in (as if slapping your hands when they aren't in line). Better versions use more dimensions so that there is forward and back as well as out and in.

In my group classes, I have chosen in recent years to concentrate on those postures that are repeated most often in the slow form to narrow the number of techniques covered a few times a week to manageable levels—as opposed to trying to get even a meager understanding of the full 37 distinct postures. And I have not always picked the easiest application possible for each posture, as you can learn a lot by trying to do things the hard way.

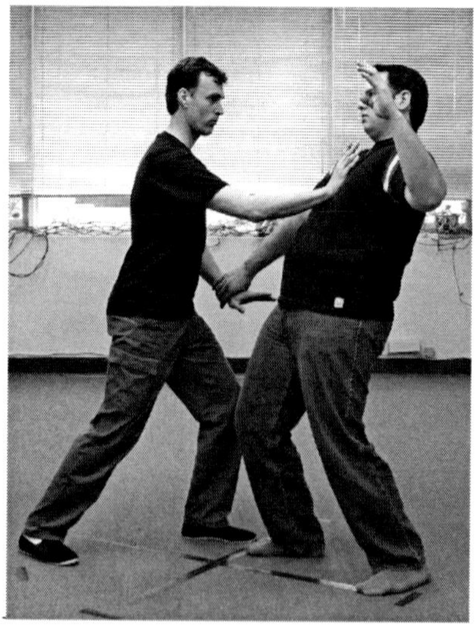

In fact, this is recognized as being the preferred route in many traditional taiji schools. You spend months and years contorting yourself and practicing difficult ways of doing things to broaden your skill levels.

Cal moves forward to strike with the final portion of brush knee.

Once the teacher thinks you are ready, you learn to do the martial stuff in a different way that seems considerably easier.

Kicks tend to be focused on the bladder area or the kidneys at the highest in practical terms and are more often aimed at the knees or ankles (and even at the hip-joint) as a way of doing what is called "breaking the root" of the opponent. Such offensive use of the legs normally supports or follows what the hands are doing and, in general, is used either to bring the opponent's attention downward while you attack high, or to follow up a striking technique while your opponent is distracted high.

Low kicks can also be useful for jamming someone's footwork, although Yang stylists are often told not to kick or knee (e.g., golden rooster stands on right leg) unless they are very sure of their balance and timing and preferably have already grabbed or struck the opponent with their hands.

While there are always exceptions to the rule, I don't think that high kicking should be your first weapon of choice unless you kick low first to set up the high kick and your opponent has less skill than you. If high kicking were as good for fighting as it is sometimes held up to be, there would not be rules in some kickboxing competitions that enforce kicking a certain number of times per round as compared to the number of punches thrown.

Nor would there be rules in MMA and Thai Boxing competitions limiting the use of what is often referred to as "plowing," in which one athlete grabs the attacking leg after evading or blocking a high kick and then uses that leg as a lever to move the attacker backward until he or she falls over—a tactic that is very effective on the street.

Two: The Fast or Sparring Set (Large San Sau)

While it is certainly not wrong to practice the long, slow form at a quicker pace for a variety of reasons, it is a mistake to think that the fast form is the slow form done more quickly (as some unscrupulous teachers have claimed). The real Yang style fast form is completely different from the long, slow form and is getting harder and harder to find, even in China, although in recent years a modern version has been created as part of the overall reformation of the traditional martial arts by the China Sport Committees and colleges.

The traditional set does not come from the Chen style and seems unique to the Yang tradition. The origins of this form are sketchy as, for a long time, it was considered secret training and those who learned it were told to deny that it even existed. From what I have seen, there is no common agreement as to who invented it, but either Yang Ban Hou or Yang Shao Hou (or both) are the most likely sources.

To confuse the issue even further, some of the modern standard bearers in the Yang family have stated publicly that this form is not a legitimate part of their curriculum, as it was not invented by a Yang family member, and that such training is not necessary. A cynic might see this as an implication that it was probably created somewhere along the line by a senior student who wasn't a family member.

However you approach its lineage, this two-person sequence is a work of art and it is worth the effort in North America to seek out those rare teachers and their affiliate instructors who can teach you a competent version of this training tool. I learned and practiced the set taught by Erle Montaigue and have seen those taught by Dr. Yang Jwing-ming in the United States and Sam Masich in Canada. All are worth the effort of pursuing if you are serious about your Yang-style martial training. I am sure that there are other good versions available here and there, but many of the Yang-style teachers that you meet, even the Chinese ones, have never heard of this form, much less practice or teach it.

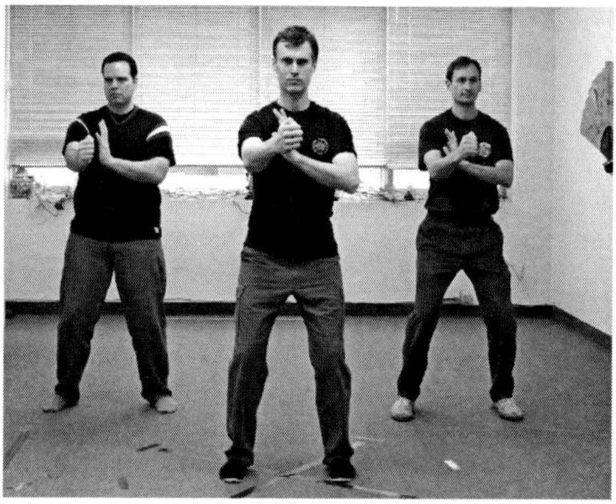

Shown here are the first several postures of the "A," or attacking side of the solo version of the fast or sparring set (large san sau). This is a wonderful old martial exercise that not many people get the chance to see.

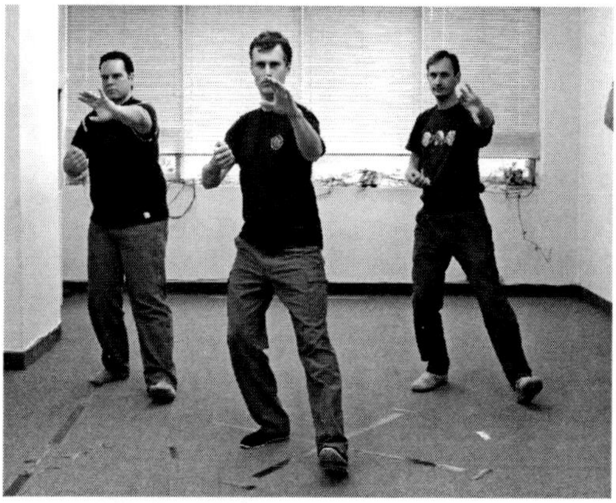

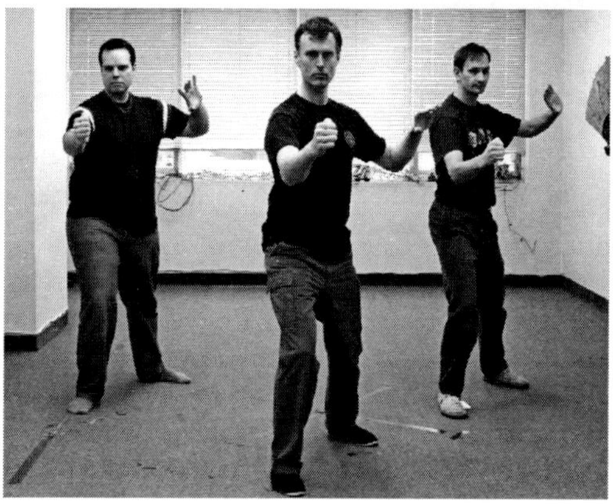

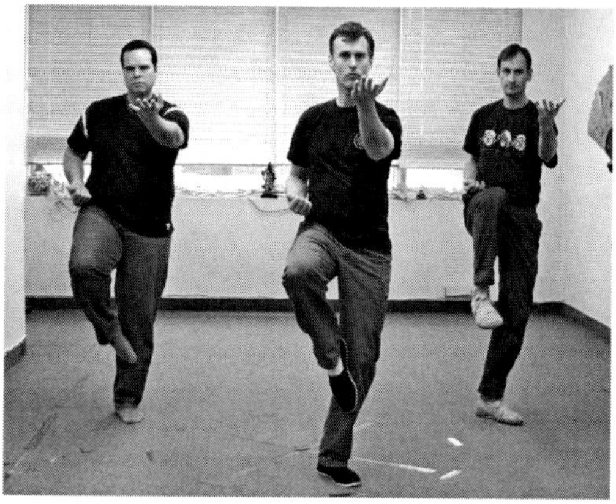

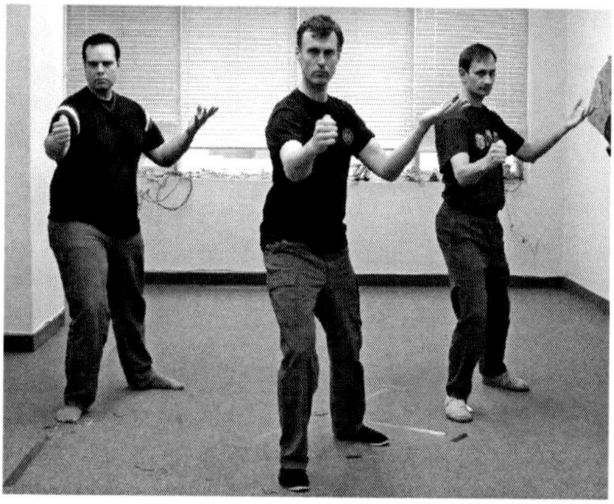

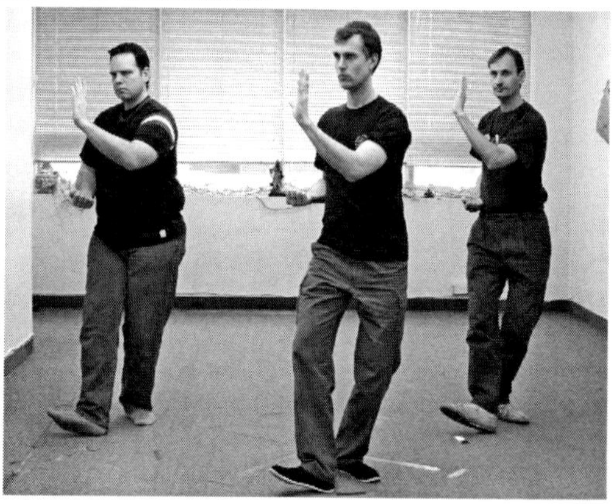

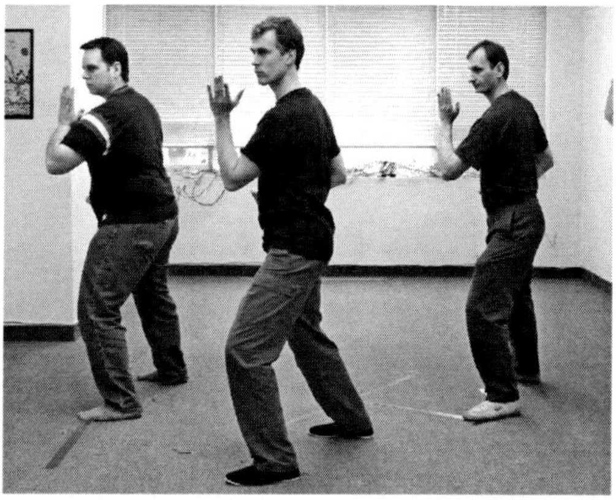

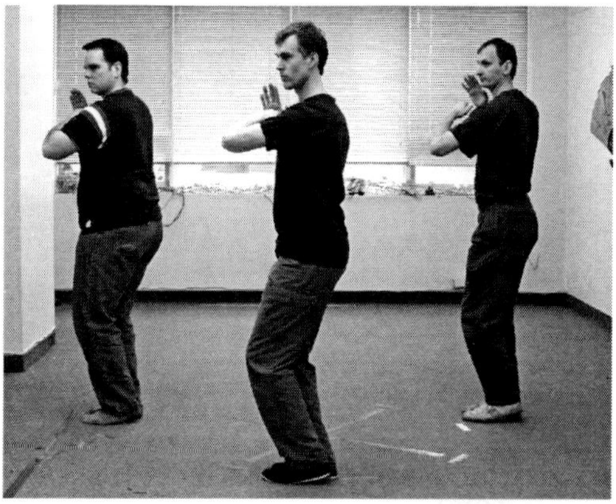

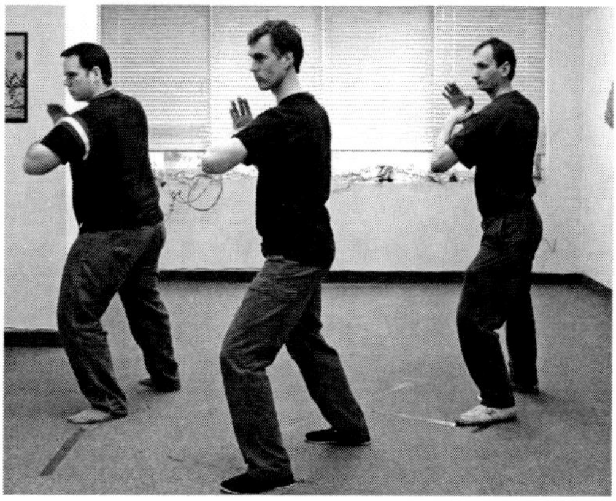

It is true that some of the martial techniques are museum pieces in that no one is likely to attack you with old-style tactics like slant flying. However, maintaining your balance and aplomb for the few minutes that it will take to do one fast-paced repetition of the entire form with a partner will go a long way to teach you some valuable lessons about fighting—and semisafely to boot!

Sadly for this great training form as well as for those who would benefit from learning it, it is becoming rare partly because it takes a great deal of time to learn, a fair amount of clear space to perform, and two students who each know at least half of the solo form in order to be able to practice the application side of it.

Unfortunately some of those who still teach it, aside from the experts I just mentioned, have modified it for a variety of reasons, including making it easier to teach and safer to practice for the general Yang-style student. This is done partly out of concern for older, out-of-shape students and partly because of legal liability issues. For example, I have seen it done by students of one late master in which the two players never actually even made contact with each other while doing the application side of the set. They each did their own thing at a safe distance from each other, so that it became a synchronized taiji-like dance—sensitivity and choreography at the expense of martial realism

Of course, it is important to be careful while training for a variety of reasons and you must, in some ways, do the interaction incorrectly for your partner's safety unless both participants are of equal size and skill—incorrectly in the sense of not going too fast or using explosive energy. At this level, the form teaches you which technique counters which technique and also lets you get used to a certain amount of contact with your partner who, in theory, knows what is coming next.

In the end, the true prizes of such long-term training are improved martial timing, distance, and contact appreciation, and using effective yielding and counterattacking as well as developing a sense of peripheral vision and martial intention, rather than the individual techniques themselves.

Pay attention to the following points when beginning the study of any competent version of this form with a partner:

- Many of the defensive methods will only work easily when you learn to move into an incoming force in a diagonal manner, or move away from the incoming force only as much as necessary rather than "running away" from it.
- Whenever you lift a knee, remember to round the crotch and face the sole of the hanging foot into your supporting knee, but do not place your foot on the knee. This emptying process does not mean that you need to lift the knee high (unless it is meant to be a knee strike), but rather that you lift it sufficiently for it to be easy to reposition as necessary and so that you can more easily drop all of your body weight into the next technique.
- Whenever your feet are together, you should look double-weighted *but not be that way*. The combative idea is to try and deceive your opponent so that he or she doesn't know for sure which direction your next step will be (even though your sparring partner should) as your feet are not always placed obviously in relation to your weighting.
- Most of what seem to be pulling movements on the wrists of your partner are really backward and downward jerking or plucking actions. My friend and mentor, Erle Montaigue, calls doing this a "negative strike," but most who try to do so don't have the authority he brings to bear when he does this. Be very careful when training, as you can cause whiplash (the whole idea in

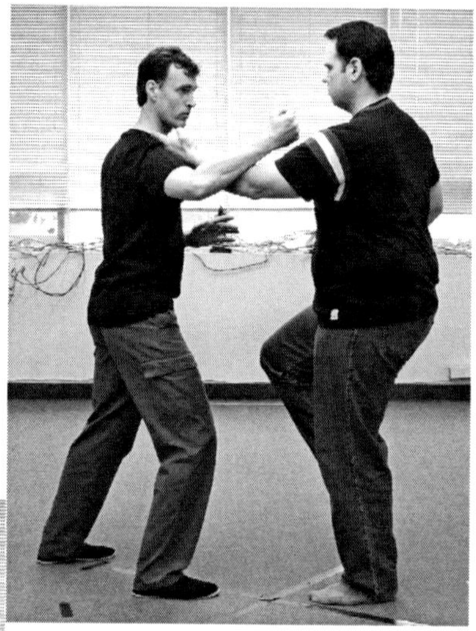

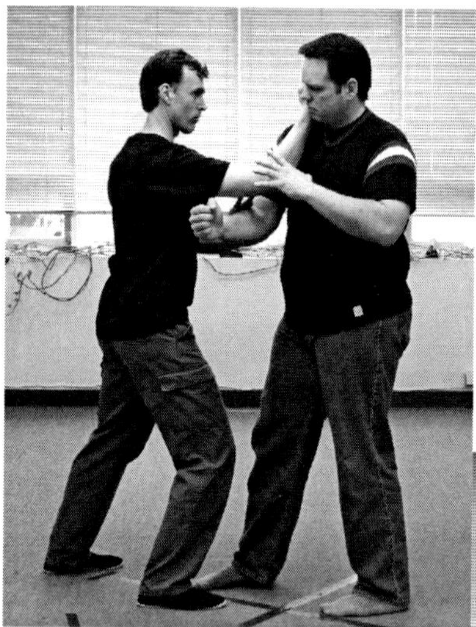

Cal does the "B," or defending side of the set with Mike.

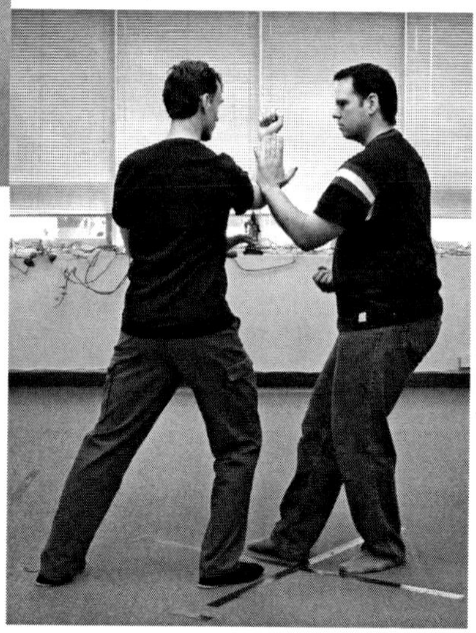

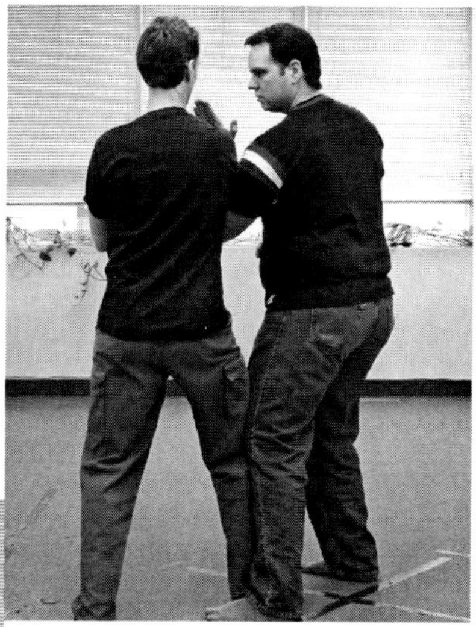

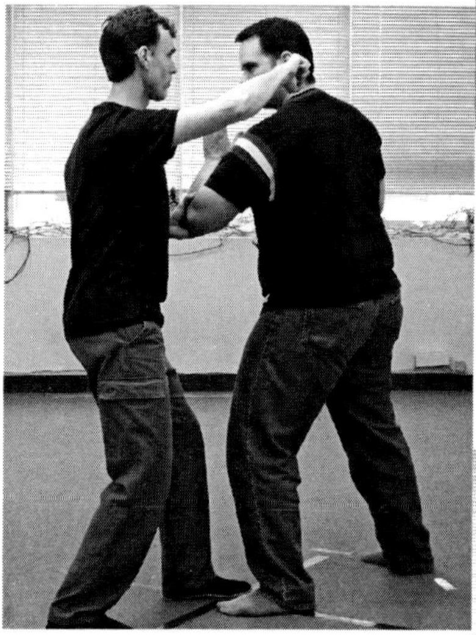

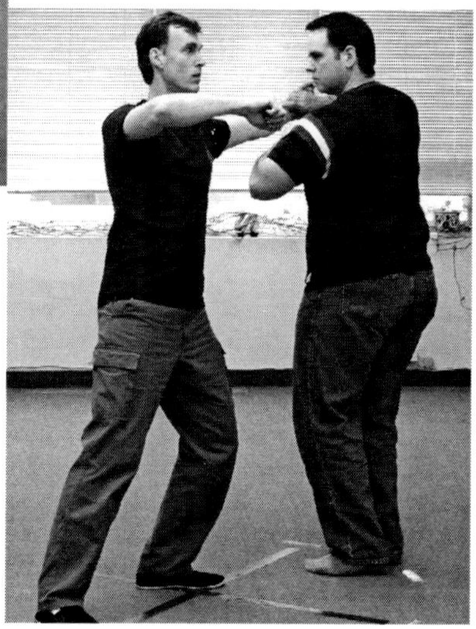

a martial sense) if you do it too much and your training partner reacts stiffly or can't get his or her wrist free at the right time.

- Learning how to get your wrist or elbow free—the right way—is one of the key skills that you can learn from the practice of the interactive side of this two-person form. Never let anyone hold on to your wrist or elbow in a martial context. You are giving them too much potential control, not only of that arm, but of the balance in your upper body as well if they have any grappling or throwing skills.
- Learn the individual techniques and interactive modules by counting them as "one" for the defensive aspect, then "two" for the offensive aspect, but remember that the majority are really one action when done well or explosively—and a few are always a one-count right from the beginning.
- Verbalizing can help you to exhale through the mouth and do reverse breathing to power your fajing strikes. However, don't do it too loudly, as you may use more speed than you wanted to strike your partner.

Two-person sets act as a martial bridge for many students to bring them to the edge of spontaneity in a martial sense. Spontaneity is essential in a good martial athlete or sportsman of any kind. This kind of skill is usually born from considerable experience as well as tactical skill, though it doesn't hurt to have some genetic aptitude. Many practitioners never seem able to get "out of the box" in terms of how they react to anything that they haven't experienced in a formal training session in their style.

Lack of the ability to be spontaneous in one's martial movement is very common in modern martial disciplines that rely too much on techniques and forms and not enough on basic training as well as principles of movement and posture.

If two-person sets become a choreography, even a fast and furious one, then the martial lessons to be learned tend to be superficial. Real fights seldom last a long time, despite what you see in the movies; one fast round of this form only takes a couple of minutes and thus lasts longer than the average real street confrontation. Only when well-trained and conditioned martial athletes are involved do contests last for round after round.

Of course, this does not mean that you shouldn't have the strength and stamina to go longer, but a street fight doesn't necessarily last all that long for a variety of reasons (e.g., witnesses interfering, police arriving, one person being severely overmatched from the beginning, etc.).

Finally, I have always found it interesting in my own students that those who take most naturally to free-sparring of any kind sometimes have the least patience or aptitude for structured two-person exercises. On the other hand, most modern students seem to need the structure to make progress, even though some of these will also have trouble transcending it.

Particularly for those who don't have a lot of relevant martial experience, large san sau can be a valuable addition to your long, slow practice, even if you only practice the solo version, in that it does benefit the cardiovascular system in Western terms—yang to complement the yin of the long, slow form, which does not challenge that system in the same way.

By the way, there is no consensus of opinion on how this form should be taught. I learned it as a long solo form that can be split in two and practiced with a partner who each does a half. Others only teach it as an interactive exercise and never encourage the students to do it solo, while still others teach the solo version only to senior students. Some old-timers even insist that this set doesn't exist and teach it as a "secret" to only a few students.

Three: Push-Hands (Tui Shou)

Push-hands include a wide variety of formal two-person exercises that are designed to refine the ability of the student to use four of the eight energies that are often considered the core of the Yang style as a martial system. By the way, these four energies—ward-off (peng), rollback (lu), press (ji), and push (an)—are not simply techniques. They are methods of generating power in that peng can be described as a whole-body force moving forward and upward, lu is a whole-body force moving downward and to one side, ji (sometimes called "squeeze" in English) is a whole-body force moving forward and downward, while an (sometimes called "press forward") is a whole-body force moving first downward and then releasing upward and away.

The formal training methods of push-hands (also sometimes called in English "four hands" or "joining hands" or, in older Chinese texts, "striking hands") teach the interaction of the four energies as discussed earlier in the sense that one leads naturally into its partner method as a follow-up technique, For example, rollback is a natural follow-up to ward-off if the other person grabs your right hand, or one method can also be used to cancel out its partner. For example, you can use press to cancel rollback if the latter is not skillfully applied.

Different teachers will usually focus on one or two methods of push-hands and will emphasize the ones that they do best or did best when younger or found the most versatile for fighting (if they were fighters), or the ones that were easiest to teach in a group format (if they are lazy or have lazy students). Even today there are many valid approaches to formal push-hands methods, even within the Yang style, much less when you cross into the other family styles.

Unfortunately, for those students hoping that there is uniformity of opinion on which method is the best, there are so many varied ways to exploit body mechanics that many

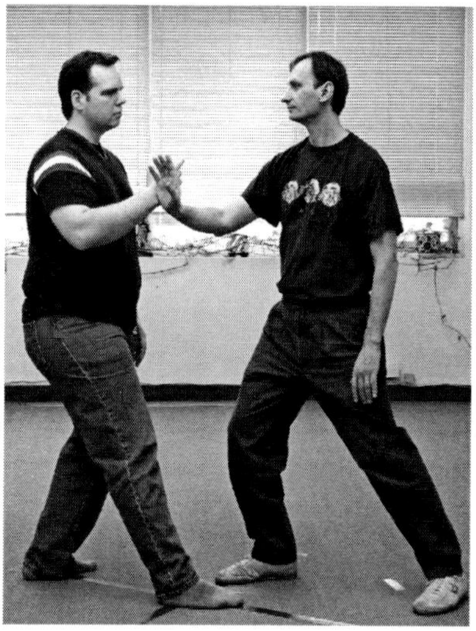

While performing single push-hands, Mike sits back and uses his spine to turn and deflect an incoming force through his arm, then counterattacks with his palm. But Alan is ready and also uses peng to set up his next move. Thus the exercise can be done back and forth for a variety of training purposes.

teachers will, consciously or otherwise, choose to emphasize the things that they do best. So it can be difficult for the students used to one teacher's approach to work with someone who uses a different power, much less cope with the intricacies of detail that often differentiate one push-hands method from another.

Furthermore, a heavier, taller teacher will emphasize the methods that work for him and a shorter, lighter teacher will emphasize the skills that work for him. Students will adapt, or fail to adapt, to this according - to their aptitude and effort. Sometimes a more enlightened teacher will attempt to teach a variety of approaches (e.g., diagonal power, vertical power, horizontal power, or blending at least two out of three). Most often, one such dimension is emphasized.

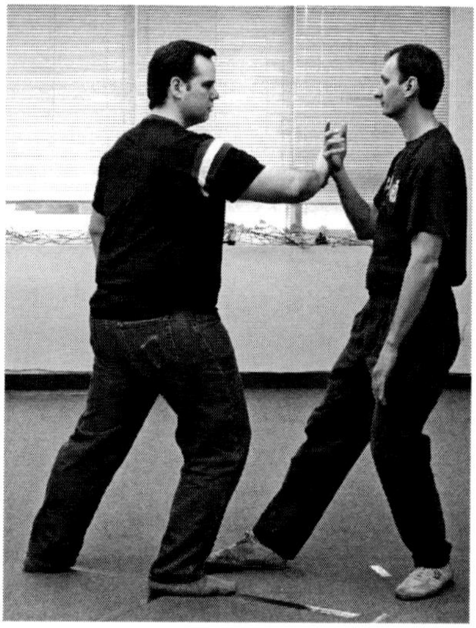

Sadly, many modern versions of push-hands have become overly sani-

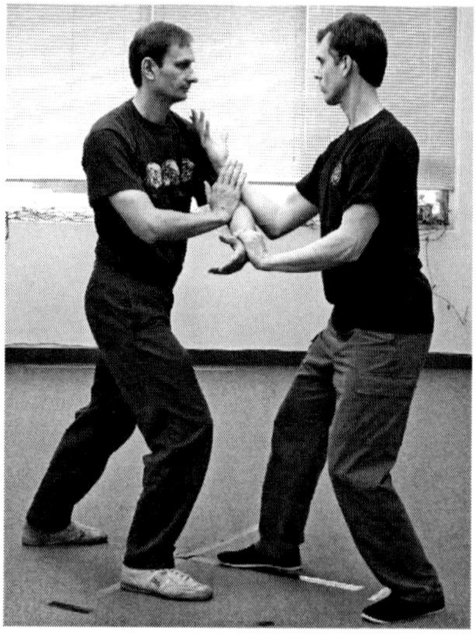

During double push-hands training, Cal tries to apply rollback to Alan's arm. Among other possible applications, this could be a way of jerking on the wrist to straighten the elbow to make it more vulnerable to being struck, or it can be a way of having neutralized Alan's previous attempt to apply ward-off offensively. Alan uses his right hand to neutralize Cal's attempt and to set up his own follow-up move.

tized to make them safer to practice in a large group setting or for competitive purposes. Today, instead of training sensitivity to a partner's gross and subtle body movements as a prelude to being able to affect their balance negatively as you counterattack in a variety of ways, such exercises all too often degenerate either into competitive struggling or going through the motions a little too cooperatively while the participants simultaneously discuss who won the latest football game.

Having said that, it is also true for the highly skilled that it is possible to do lively push-hands without seeming to pay conscious attention, as with proper training your body can learn to do a variety of martial skills under pressure more or less automatically. One of my former instructors, Allan Weiss, used to relate how his teacher, the late Lee Shiu Pak, who had trained in Shanghai under Chen Wei Ming, would do vigorous push-hands with Allan and the other senior students while holding a lighted cigarette casually in one hand as he easily fended off their frantic attacks with the other.

By contrast, the average modern taiji practitioner has never been in a fight in his or her adult life, and has neither the combative background nor the emotional inclination, much less the physical health and strength, to really learn anything valid solely from push-hands. This is often true no matter how efficient the training methods may be or have been. If some of the raw materials are missing when you refine anything, you won't get the final product that you desire and expect.

I think that too many Westerners get confused by seeing push-hands done by the few experts that are still around. It looks easy and those watching assume that the exercises within push-hands are the crucial element in skill development, forgetting about all the years of getting bruised, battered, and sweaty while learning martial basics.

In the beginning it is essential to train with someone you trust who has more skill at push-hands than you do. This is less important in applications work, as you can at least tell, objectively, if the method works in some way since your tactics will keep you from getting touched, hit, or knocked over. If you have a partner who doesn't understand it better than you, then the two of you may eventually be able to move in a coordinated manner and make it "look good" on a superficial level, but there's a big difference between how it looks to a casual observer and how it is as an effective martial training method.

To make it worse, many modern practitioners focus on New Age push-hands games that are more useful in getting older middle-class adults in satin outfits to part with their money in return for gaining the illusion of having done taiji as a martial art. I don't mean to sound harsh about this, as doing push-hands with a good partner can be fun as well as challenging, but not if both haven't got core combative skills.

Whatever pattern you practice, most mainstream variations use the forward bow stance by preference, and there are a few generalities that should be observed, no matter what interpretation your instructor or style follows. For example, the legs must be (or grow) strong, as they must not only support your body weight but must shift smoothly in time with your partner's weight changes. In the long run, you learn to do the appropriate tactics both from a stationary position and while stepping in a variety of formal patterns that can involve stepping once, stepping three times, walking in circles, or freestyle movement. Some styles and teachers emphasize at an advanced stage of learning to move the feet so subtly and constantly that a less skillful partner doesn't even know that you are creeping up on them until it is too late.

Competent push-hands also demands that your body mechanics are structurally sound. For example, the ankles and knees are not meant to rotate, except minimally when you shift or step forward and backward. As in form practice, one way of ensuring that your legs are structurally aligned is to ensure that the knees don't bend farther than the tips of the toes of their respective feet and that your lower leg stays relatively vertical. This applies whether you are moving your weight onto the front or rear leg when changing from a bow to a back-sitting stance, which are the postures most commonly used in structured push-hands methods.

In addition, the torso must be relaxed and supple so that it can direct the energy from the feet to the hands. Some versions of the Yang style will also advocate that you must learn to differentiate between the waist and the hips as well. Sometimes, the hips and shoulders will move strictly as a unit. At other times a subtle or exaggerated (depending on the teacher's preferences) twisting or untwisting of the trunk between the last ribs and the hip bones will add power to the turning or striking.

As in all aspects of training, the spine must be erect with the top of the head lifted and the chin lightly tucked in so as to keep all the body's energy and physical centers aligned. Keeping the spine straight and the buttocks relaxed connects the hands(s) being used to the rear or front foot, as is necessary in terms of the potential for power generation.

The shoulders must relax and not hunch upward with muscular effort. This is particularly important when receiving force, as raising the shoulders will likely upset your balance even if you can prevent the incoming force from making contact. This is most likely to happen if you lift the "active" elbow unnecessarily high.

Speaking of which, the elbows must stay slightly bent and relaxed, only rising momentarily to be able to open as a prelude to a closing action that follows while practicing issuing energy as a push or a strike. Doing so excessively opens the ribs and kidneys to the tactics of a skillful opponent. The forearms must learn to coordinate, under pressure, with the movement of the elbows as well as the shoulders so that twisting when gripping another wrist and elbow is not just a gross attempt to gain leverage by jerking the arms forcefully with your shoulder muscles and biceps and triceps.

In the same way that you must avoid being double-weighted in the legs, the wrists must always be changing from one state to another (i.e., you never have both hands yin or both hands yang at exactly the same time). This is partly so that you can add the force of the hand opening and stretching to a palm strike, and partly so that you can release your own grip on the other person smoothly and instantly if such is necessary. Having supple wrists helps the hands become sensitized to those subtle physical movements in your partner's limb that signal a change of direction or force as—or, with enough skill, before—they occur.

Similarly, while contact with your partner's limbs is essential, it should not become a case of simply sticking for the sake of sticking. A skillful opponent will lure you into paying too much attention to one arm so that he or she can attack you suddenly with the other. You have to be able to connect and disconnect smoothly and in a supple manner while doing push-hands, otherwise your skills will never rise above a basic level.

This is based on a sensitivity that allows the experienced practitioner to feel the opponent's balance and force, while simultaneously adjusting his own balance and force accordingly to obtain or maintain an advantageous position. To put it simply, each hand has to be able to grab suddenly and effectively or open just as instantly, if necessary. Doing this under any kind of martial pressure is much harder than most beginners assume.

In many ways, single push-hands is harder to do than double push-hands and stationary methods are easier to practice than moving ones—even those that are heavily choreographed. Doing push-hands while moving your feet can teach you how to get your feet away from someone trying to step on or trap them while keeping your hands busy. It can also begin teaching you how to follow another person's timing, as learning how to follow is often the first step in learning how to lead, or impose your own timing on someone in a martial sense.

Conversely, push-hands easily degenerates into being done so sensitively and lightly as too make it hard to evaluate whether or not you are doing it or just going through the motions. However, it is also true that such methods don't have to have the brutal nature of the old Yang training. Erle Montaigue relates what one of his Chinese teachers told him about studying with the Yang Shao Hou: "Sometimes bones were broken and I often went home with blood on my vest." Push-hands can remain civilized and still be an effective learning tool, but you shouldn't take it too far the other way.

Speaking of fooling yourself, some teachers I have met advocate the value of practicing push-hands patterns by yourself, but it is difficult to believe that this could sharpen your yielding, neutralizing, or sensitivity skills past a very basic level. Along these lines, I once visited a taiji school in which a room full of overweight middle-aged people were all earnestly practicing repetitions of double push-hands by themselves in rows. The instructor told me that this was the ideal way for them to train, as they could visualize martial training while doing so without running the risk of injury. "After all," he told me rather smugly, "the mind is everything in taiji."

I hate to contradict someone who was teaching many more students than I usually have at any given time, but while the role of the mind is essential in training intelligently, it is hardly "everything." By contrast, a good Western boxer shadowboxes in front of a mirror to practice certain combinations and work on his posture and body mechanics—not to learn how to fight.

If I may offer a few clues to developing push-hands skill, they would be:

- Practice with a variety of partners in terms of body weight, heights, and skill. Each type of body build has its own advantages and disadvantages. You can only learn this by practicing with a variety of people.
- Practice with both a light and heavy intensity, as the former can aid in developing speed while the latter can aid in developing "connectivity" in terms of using all parts of the body in a synchronized and coordinated manner.
- Vary the speed between slow and fast so that you get used to being able to flow and change directions at a variety of speeds.
- Remember to help each other learn by not working too much beyond each partner's abilities, otherwise it tends to turn into the childish equivalent of "Take that!" and "Oh yeah, you're gonna get it now!"

More experienced students can practice chi sau and san sau. The Chinese characters for the former mean literally "sticky hands," while those for the latter mean "free hands." These are less structured methods of push-hands and the idea is to use a variety of methods and footwork to successfully attack and defend while always keeping at least one hand in contact with your partner's arm(s). These ways of training go about as far as push-hands can go toward being a fast and spontaneous way of practicing attacking and defending, although even this has limitations in the sense that you are starting in contact with your training partner.

When done by two skillful partners who are not too dissimilar in size, the speed and intensity can approach real fighting without being too dangerous. In fact, it is as close to free sparring as many traditional taijiquan schools will go. With intermediate level students, I suggest doing it as a a fixed-step choreography in which each person learns to shift in coordination with their partner's movements, while attempting to remain in contact with each other's forearms during the two basic patterns that use brush knee, wave hands, and neutralize to push.

Remember always to go back to circling the arms after each successful attack or defense, or switch smoothly from one type of structured push-hands to another and back to chi sau. For more advanced practitioners, these are useful as moving "almost anything goes" exercises in which each partner attempts to strike and control the other while remaining in meaningful contact with each other through the arms.

In the beginning, don't use kicks and only use light contact on your intended target to score. Eventually, you can use kicks, grappling, and full contact to the torso, if you have a padded floor, the requisite falling skills, and a tough skin.

It has been my experience that those students who excel at these training methods are not always those who enjoyed the more basic push-hands methods. In fact, quite often it is the opposite. Those who naturally take to freestyle push-hands are those who don't like or relate as easily to structured push-hands. I also suspect that those who take to them most easily are those who have some previous experience in rougher forms of martial play.

It will probably take many months before your body can respond instantly and spontaneously to your partner's attempts to penetrate your defenses—even in a relatively slow and civilized manner. This brings up the other problem with modern push-hands: Progress will probably come more quickly with daily practice, assuming you have some aptitude and good partners.

So don't be surprised if it takes a while when you only get the chance to practice with a partner once or twice a week. Remember that such training can be tedious if you don't have a good training partner—and that cuts both ways—so keep that in mind when trying to deal with your partner's efforts.

Four: Large Pull-Down (Da Lu)

This exercise is also often called "big pull-down" in English and is a structured method of practicing the other four core Yang martial energies: pluck (cai), rend (lie), elbow (zhou), and shoulder stroke (kao), effectively. These are said to correspond to the diagonal points on the compass and understanding this on some level is usually the point at which a student starts to realize that the traditional concept of the five directions is more profound than they were led to believe.

The five directions are traditionally described in English as advance (jin), retreat (tui), look left (zuo gu), look right (you pan), and central equilibrium (zhong din). The first four are partly about those cardinal directions and how to exploit them martially, and are partly hints on how important it is to

In practicing da lu, Cal pulls/jerks Alan by the arm while doing pluck, but Alan goes with the downward pressure to start freeing his arm from Cal's grip. He steps in preparation for striking Cal's chest with either his elbow or his shoulder.

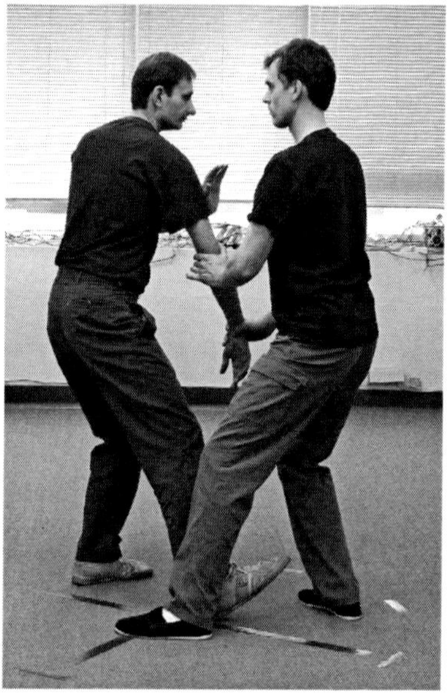

be able to move freely and not just be rooted to the spot—no matter how well you may be able to relax.

The fifth direction is said to be the most essential concept, even though to Western eyes it seems to describe a lack of movement as being a crucial form of movement—which certainly seems contradictory in the very least. I won't try to describe what it really means, partly because I no longer believe in spoon-feeding any serious student of taijiquan. Let me just tease you with the suggestion that the real source of any balanced and efficient martial movement is turning your spine into a central axis that can move freely in any direction as the moment and the situation demands.

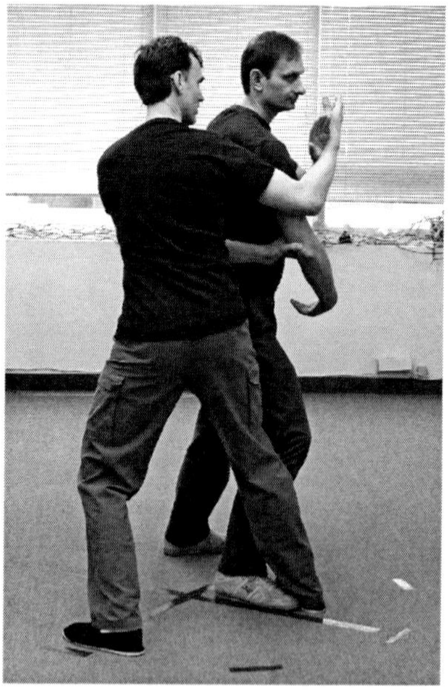

Some teachers talk about "finding the square in the circle" as well as "finding the circle in the square"

Cal moves out of the way at the last moment and executes rend to control Alan's lead foot and elbow while attempting to strike Alan on the left side of his neck or head with his free hand.

when describing the subtle purposes behind practicing da lu. This concept refers to finding the power in the martial relationships between the diagonal and cardinal points on a compass. Many forms of da lu will actually use some version of such a representational diagram painted or scraped into the ground where that method is practiced.

Da lu also trains the student to "cut the corners" instead of either moving away too far to one side or retreating or attacking too directly unless you are sure that you can just overpower the attacker in terms of brute force. The latter approach is hardly ideal from an internal perspective, although I often tell my students that it is better to succeed at defending yourself crudely than to stick to your principals—when such are still only theoretical skills—so much that you end up with your face in the dust.

Defending properly often requires that you wait a little and use superior timing rather than jumping the gun and walking into a feint. By the way, in some styles, da lu is the first training method to start teaching more experienced beginners the concept of bridging the gap that usually exists initially between them and an attacker and his target as well as evasion skills.

As with all aspects of training in the Yang styles and Yang family, there are a variety of formal ways of practicing da lu. I have learned three distinct methods over the years from teachers and have seen several others demonstrated. To be useful in a martial sense, any variation that you learn must have some speed and close-range contact with your training partners, otherwise it is almost impossible to learn the valuable lessons that this method can bring.

As far as I am concerned, two of the most important aspects of this exercise occur in the first two exchanges—if your partner pulls his or her wrist free or resists with skill or superior size when you begin pluck, remember to do your follow-up method of rend as a counterattack rather than as a defense. Doing this smoothly and as an aspect of "push-pull" training is very disconcerting to the person who thinks that they have gotten free of you. Just be careful that you don't hit your partner more than you want to while doing so.

In the beginning, practice with someone roughly of the same size. Significant height differences can make some of the methods problematic. For example, when practicing with someone taller than you, be careful of your knees, as his kneecap is liable to strike vulnerable points on the sides of your legs when he steps in to do a shoulder strike.

Five: Traditional Weapons Forms and Martial Function

The most commonly found traditional weapons in the Yang style are the single-edged curved broadsword, the double-edged straight sword, the long spear that is 6 to 9 feet in length (sometimes even longer), and the staff that can vary in length from roughly 4 to 8 feet. These are normally fashioned from rattan, waxwood, or hardwood.

While the traditional weapons have little functional role in self-defense in a world of guns and weapons of mass destruction, they are important tools for refining your understanding of unarmed training. In the old days, you were expected not only to be proficient in at least one of these weapons, but also to have some idea of how each of the weapons you were liable to have to fight against would function in the hands of a skilled opponent.

Modern training with such martial tools can also be a lot of "fun" for those so inclined. Many years ago, I was at a week-long training camp and the organizer, Sam Masich, was missing at lunchtime while the rest of us were eating and relaxing after a grueling morning of practice. His girlfriend was going around asking where he was and was finally told by someone that, instead of resting and eating, he was trying to learn some new techniques with rattan staffs from one of the participants who knew something about stick techniques from another oriental system. She gave the kind of sigh that only an exasperated woman can muster and muttered, "Men are such little boys as soon as they get their hands on a stick!"

Aside from being interesting ways to vary your training, the characteristics of each weapon help to develop the body in ways that are not often easily accomplished through empty-hand forms and exercises. The extra weight can build arm as well as upper body strength. In addition, holding a weapon in one or both hands changes the ways in which you balance and move. This necessitates a heightened sense of awareness of your body and the space through which you and the weapon are moving. You have to learn not only to control your body and the six dimensions of movement as well as the five directions, but also extend that to the weapon moving forward and back, up and down, as well as side to side.

This is hard enough to achieve when practicing by yourself, but these new skills become even more crucial when you are trying to be attentive of someone else who is trying to use a weapon against you, even when it is only relatively cooperative two-person training.

One of the greatest benefits of training with any weapon is learning how the shape and structure of each weapon affects, determines, and limits its martial function. While all weapons share similarities within their broad categories—long or short, edged or impact—each has special attributes and limitations that you must get accustomed to. It is also true that all weapons are the same in the sense that they are best used by a skillful practitioner whose skills have become such that he or she could literally pick up any item and use it as an improvised weapon in an emergency. Some Chinese hard styles have bench, fan, and chopstick forms for this very practical reason.

One of the most difficult aspects of learning the basics of traditional weapon use is learning how to hold each weapon with just the right amount of muscular force. Even some relatively skillful practitioners will discover that they are not as relaxed or as strong as they thought when trying to master the correct grip with the required flexibility of wrist and elbow. It is also true that much of the difficulty in learning to hold a weapon properly comes from developing the proper grip using only the thumb and one or two fingers, rather than clenching all the fingers around the handle or shaft as untrained common sense might argue.

There are different theories as to which fingers should be used, and the best way to discover what works best for you is to experiment with a variety of grips while training with a partner. The goal is to have a grip flexible enough to allow you to manipulate the weapon easily within its functional ranges, while still retaining the strength to absorb an impact without losing your grip on the weapon. It is not easy to learn this and you won't if you never train with a partner and actually practice a variety of applications.

I firmly believe that intermediate and advanced practitioners should, for all the reasons just discussed, develop a minimal understanding of the solo form and martial usage for at least one of the following weapons and to have some comprehension of the main characteristics of usage for the others.

The Broadsword/Saber

First of all, it is important to differentiate between the two different weapons that are often called indiscriminately in English "saber" and "broadsword." The Yang family saber more properly refers to the long, slightly-curved single-edged weapon that Yang Cheng-fu used in his later years. In one story of how this tradition started, he received a a European cavalry saber as a gift and he liked the feel of the blade so much that he had a traditional Chinese guard and handle

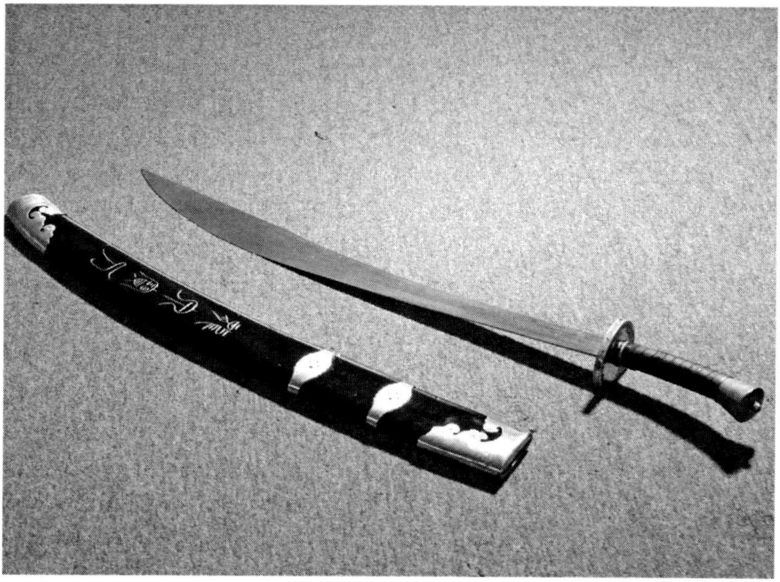

A modern copy of a Yang-style broadsword.

mounted on the blade. In another version of the story, it was a Japanese katana blade that he had mounted in a more Chinese manner.

Modern copies of these are available and many Yang stylists have started to practice with it exclusively—and not always appropriately, if their style actually uses a Yang style form designed for the more common broadsword.

The Yang-style broadsword is the traditional Chinese dao (knife) whose single edged blade is thicker, wider, and shorter in length when compared to the weapon used by Yang Cheng-fu and most who follow the Yang family lineage. It is also heavier at the tip of the blade so that its balance is quite different from the aforementioned saber. It also can have a short but sharp edge on the topside of the blade near the tip, making it useful for slicing upward at short range—which is the preferred range for this weapon.

There's a valuable dictum that states: "form dictates usage; usage dictates form." Consequently, the weight, balance, and function of the weapon that you use should certainly dictate the structure and the body mechanics of any form that is designed to allow you to mimic using that weapon.

This perhaps explains why the forms that used only the traditional broadsword, where the emphasis was the weight of the tip of the weapon for slashing or chopping, are different from those using the saber, as the latter is a finer, more evenly balanced weapon capable of more finesse in its cutting, as well as being more versatile as a thrusting tool that the dao.

Aside from this, it is very difficult to explain in objective terms how the same form from the same source could end up being so different, but I think it is also yet another example of how forms and methods tend to differ depending on the skills, experience, weapon used, as well as body types and preferences of those teaching them. It is also true that, quite often, solo forms end up looking and being different because the person demonstrating hasn't learned the original form properly.

Within reason, I think this is another good example of why you shouldn't obsess about which Yang style form is best and which expert is most correct, as taiji—and, for that matter, life —is rarely that cut and dried. In terms of training needs, the problem is amassing enough skill and experience to be able to know what suits your physique, skills, and personality, and is still true to the principles of the discipline.

Practicing with either version of this weapon can teach you about extending your reach and force to the tip as well as the edge of the weapon and, as it (usually) only has one sharp edge, it's a little safer to do so when you first start exploring weapons. Please note that I didn't say better—I said safer.

This weapon is sometimes described as having a Yang nature and it certainly is a challenge to use it properly even when moving slowly when compared the the fast and furious pace favored by the harder styles. The bold, twisting, wide-swinging tactics of either version of this weapon should have elegance and smoothness as well as martial effectiveness. Their use should teach you about angles and the various planes around the body.

Doing a well-structured form properly is like being inside a steel cage or at the center of a hurricane. Every stroke should cut cleanly along one of the eight cardinal directions—the square in the circle and the circle in the square. Have you figured out this taiji conundrum yet?

It is also another useful way of exploring that taiji classic (I paraphrase): "Going forward, consider backward." Particularly when dealing with the extra weight of a weapon, if you don't keep your balance when advancing, you're liable to fall over from your misguided momentum if it falls on emptiness (i.e., your target had the skill to move at the last moment). You must learn to use the weight of the saber, not depend on it to power your stroke. The strikes are chopping slices, not the rise and fall of an ax.

This is one way to learn to really relax the shoulder, elbow, and wrist without sacrificing impact and power, but it is often a rather hard way of learning to do so. Again, if you never practice actually striking a target of some kind with wooden and metal versions of this weapon, it is hard to get an appreciation of how it feels to do so.

The Staff/Spear

You may not be surprised to hear that there is a great deal of discussion in taiji circles about which is the most authentic surviving version of the staff techniques and whether or not it or the spear are actually the queen of weapons as opposed to the sword (jian), which usually gets that title.

Yang Lu-chan was, by most accounts, a master of the long spear. There are fascinating stories about his skill and dexterity with this weapon, such as being able to tear down the walls of a house quickly with it to prevent a fire in that building from spreading. In later times, his son, Yang Ban Hou, apparently ordered the metal heads removed when one of his children was accidentally killed while training with spears.

This is one version of why the staff techniques became predominant in Yang-style training. Certainly many of the staff techniques resemble those done with a spear (i.e., more thrusting movements and fewer swinging movements). It is also true that the Yang family have not retained any forms, but only teach short sequences of techniques with the longer versions of the spear and staff.

Training methods include striking various objects, including your partner's staff, to learn how to generate power from relatively short distances without having the reverberations rebound into your own hands.

Advocates of its superiority argue with conviction that the basic practices with a long staff or spear—parrying, deflecting, and thrusting—can be repeated endlessly on one's own and provide a training that builds the body and cardiovascular endurance like nothing else. Training with a spear can certainly bring you a lot of physical conditioning, but I have mixed feelings about training with this weapon. I must admit that it seems like a waste of time to spend

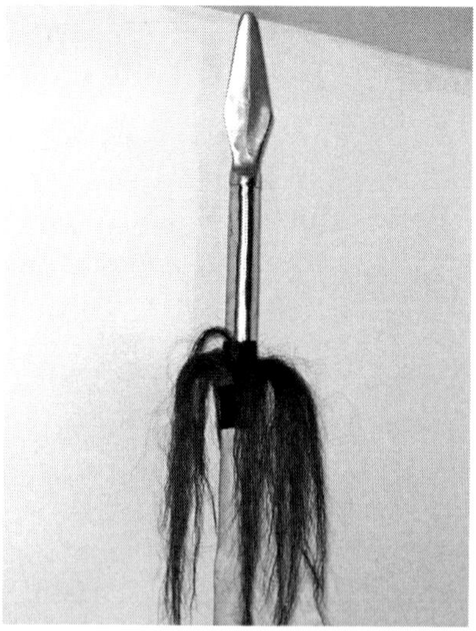

The "business end" of an 8-foot Chinese spear. Photo courtesy of Andrea Falk.

so much time practicing a weapon that really was only of use—because of its length—against mounted cavalry or formations of men armed with the same weapon and tactics.

I also suspect that a time traveler from the old days in China who had ever used a spear to save his life or earn a living would be pretty disgruntled over what he could see these days passed off as spear and staff training.

By the way, the Chinese spearhead is normally double-edged and one of the reasons that there is so much emphasis put on twisting the shaft is to aid in penetrating what you strike as well as retrieving your weapon at the end of a thrust if the target grabs the wooden shaft to try and wrestle the spear from your grip. By twisting as you withdraw, you are more likely to snatch the spear from the other person's grip and remove some or all of their fingers as the blade slides through their hands.

Chinese spears also normally have a long red fringe all the way around the base of the spearhead. This is commonly described as a way of trying to distract an opponent visually as well as providing a means of keeping any blood on the blade from easily sliding down onto the wooden shaft and making it harder for the wielder to hang onto his or her weapon.

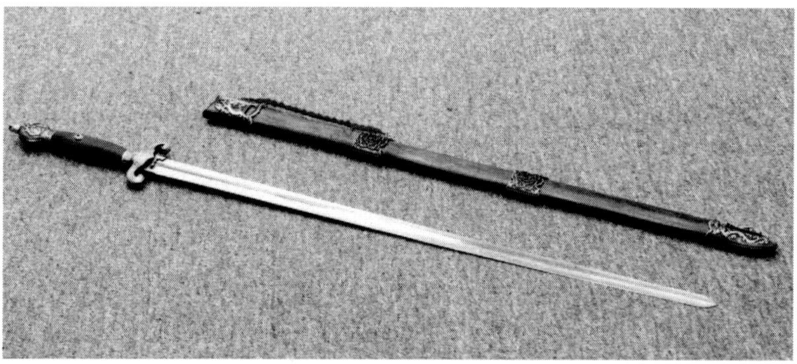

An example of a modern copy of a double-edged sword.

By contrast to the spear, the staff moves through diagonal planes around the practitioner to strike and to intimidate. Thrusting attacks using the tip of the staff move along a single line. The forward wrist is used to direct the weapon, as well as to move the forward end of the staff to parry, stick, and circle in defense and attack. Movements to the left and right or up and down are controlled by the rear hand.

Striking force is generated near the end of each posture and is a wavelike momentum developed by the practitioner's feet, waist, and spine. The wrist and shoulder may add to this force or be used to change the direction subtly if the stroke is used as a defense and followed by a thrusting action. Even without a metal spearhead, the shock of being struck by the end of a hardwood or waxwood staff is nothing that can be easily blocked, parried, or ignored.

The Straight Sword/Jian

There is a fair bit of controversy about the origins of sword usage in the Yang style. It seems fairly certain, for a variety of reasons, that it didn't come from the Chen style. As I mentioned earlier, the founder of the Yang style, Yang Lu Chan, was famous for his skill with the spear and reportedly did not teach sword.

However, his son, Ban Hou, learned the use of the sword, apparently from a Daoist monk of the Wudang Mountain (whose monks were famous for their sword skills) and became almost as well known for his swordsmanship as for his legendary harsh and taciturn nature. He taught his art to his nephew, Yang Shao Hou.

Only a few variations of Ban Hou's sword form have survived into modern times, notably that taught by Yang Jwing-ming in the United States. The only other version that I have seen was on a demonstration video by the late York Why-loo. These forms are far from identical, by any means, but they all share a structure and certain postures that don't appear in the sword forms that descend from the Yang Cheng-fu lineage.

Over the years I have learned several versions of the solo sword set attributed to Cheng-fu's lineage. All these forms share structure and postures that are common to them, although none were identical by any means. Incidentally, I have been told more than once over the years by experts that I trust that there is considerable evidence that the form taught by Cheng-fu as the Yang family solo set was actually created by one of his earlier senior students, Chen Wei Ming. This gentlemen had accumulated considerable skill with the straight sword before learning from Cheng-fu and authored a popular book on taiji sword in China in the 1920s.

Speaking of controversy, some teachers of the sword tell you that the length of the sword must be exactly tailored to your height and weight, while others say that an experienced practitioner should use the heaviest and longest sword that he can manage. It is certainly true that it can be difficult to go back to using the cheap wooden and metal swords that are normally available commercially for such practice once you have held one of the antique swords or one of the modern custom-made swords that can cost hundreds, if not thousands, of dollars—if you can find one.

On the other hand, the wooden and cheap metal weapons available today tend to splinter, break, or bend fairly easily, and it can get expensive replacing broken equipment if you practice applications—and you should.

You should consider buying the best quality metal sword that you can find and afford. Now, this is not easy in North America, as buying a sword by mail or through the Internet is not a good idea—you really need to handle any weapon before buying it to get a feel for its weight and balance. It may be a shock for those used to practicing with the swords that are easily available through martial arts stores that a good sword will have a relatively firm blade that is at least 30 inches in length, weigh 1 1/2 to 3 pounds, and have a point-of-balance as close to the hand guard as possible.

As to weight and length, I'm afraid that bigger is better when dealing with an attempt to use combat principles as opposed to wushu performance skills. That's why the people who enter competitions have weapons whose blades bend like tinfoil. The lighter the weapon, the faster they can move, and they don't have to worry about striking armor or another, better-quality sword.

As to the ornate and expensive replica weapons that have become more available across North America, even a superficial study of of the history of arms and armor will quickly reveal that function follows form (and vice-versa). Weapons that were used for fighting were normally plain and simple and the expense went into the strength and quality of the blade. Ornamental and expensively gilded, carved, or inlaid weapons were for parade functions or for officers, nobles, or royalty who usually did not actually get close to the fighting. In other words, don't buy a sword that looks like it should be displayed on your mantelpiece—that's probably all that it is good for!

Aside from the annoyance factor and the cost, It is also dangerous to use equipment that cannot hold up to even the lightest contact. I once had to pull a splinter the size and length of a wooden match out of the flesh in my right side—its entire length had been buried in me when a wooden sword brushed my side with more power than I or my training partner had expected. I have also had some nasty cuts from supposedly smooth, blunt metal edges that had been turned jagged by repeated contact.

As to the long tassels that are often seen hanging from the end of the handle of a Chinese straight sword, people whose opinion I respect have said that the tassels are useful when training solo forms, as they will wrap around your wrist, impeding your movement, if you do some of the postures incorrectly, so that the use of tassels can be thought of as a "feedback" mechanism for proper mechanics. However, on a battlefield, I would suspect that a tassel is as likely to cause your death as improve your technique. Today when taiji sword experts (a few that I have met personally and done workshops with include Yang Jwing-ming, Sam Masich, and Liang Shou-yu) demonstrate two-person applications, tassels are rarely in evidence.

In any case, the study of the sword is an interesting way of varying your practice and trying to add a new dimension to your understanding of taiji. The jian is often compared to a Chinese dragon: fast and frightening in terms of the grace and sinuous rapidity of its movement and the twisting ease with which it can "bite."

Where you would block with the broadsword, you dodge with the straight sword; where you would slam, you flick; where you would charge, you circle or sidestep. I like to think of the jian as a scalpel with a 3-foot reach, although this is not quite accurate, as a traditional weapon would have a relatively thick and blunt blade for the rear third, sometimes last half, of its length so as to be strong enough if a blocking action against a heavier weapon was needed.

Normally, the edges would be razor-sharp only near the tip, but in having two edges, the jian can cut from surprising angles and is as effective on the backstroke as on the advance. The footwork needed is nimble and developing skill with a jian is partly a matter of learning to shift, sidestep, and evade attacks as much as you parry or block them (the last tactic being reserved for martial emergencies).

To be effective, you must connect the flat of your blade (not the edge) to the opponent's and then use the weight and movement of your body to deflect his blade simultaneously and possibly affect his balance in even a small way. This should create an immediate opportunity to slice the wrist or arm that holds the sword to, literally, "disarm" him or her prior to a finishing stroke.

In unarmed combat, it is sometimes considered suitable to trade blows to the body with an opponent—if doing so gives you access to a better target, as is the strategy with "sacrifice throws" in which you fall along with the person that you have thrown, hopefully with the full weight of your body on his to increase his discomfort and minimize yours. This is not a good strategy with edged weapons. You must evade, parry, or block every attack and your opponent likewise.

Training martial function with the sword is essential in really understanding the solo aspect of your training, but even rudimentary understanding of martial usage is hard to come by in modern times. Warm-up exercises, practicing applications with a partner, and two-person sword sparring sets are all essential aspects of developing even rudimentary swordsmanship.

Most modern taiji teachers either don't understand the sword as a combat weapon or have adapted Chinese hard-style sword tactics to teach combat basics. This is not necessarily a bad thing as many stylistic purists would insist. Any form of competently taught edged-weapon training can eventually help you to understand the jian as a combative tool, even if your "stylistic purity" can suffer by such cross-training.

On the other hand, it is also true that there seems to be very little real purity in the Yang style swordsmanship that I have seen in North America, with much addition of training methods from other Chinese systems of even Western fencing—or obsessions with circling/sticking exercises that may bring some skill in sensitivity but teach nothing about combative distance and timing.

There are a few ways of telling if your teacher has some skill in swordsmanship:

- When gripping the sword handle, he does so gently but firmly with the first one or two fingers and the thumb—not the entire hand—and holds it as close to the guard as a possible. Using a tight grip is the mark of a beginner and is usually the reason that students of this weapon get sore wrists, elbows, or shoulders when they first start training with the sword. Of course, finding the right amount of pressure is not easy and many students also fall prey to using so loose a grip that they have no real control of the weapon.

- As with any aspect of good Yang style, the whole-body movement should make it seem that the sword is just an extension of the wielder's hand and that the weapons moves largely through a coordinated usage of the waist and wrist. It should not be the case of moving the body first and then using the sword by making large circular movements of the weapon primarily with the shoulder.
- A skillful swordsman can make it seem as if the sword itself leads his or her body into position—as if the weapon were pulling the person into position by the handle or even, in certain circling exercises and tactics, as if it is moving almost independently of the person holding it. I know this sounds a little silly, but you may know what I mean if you ever get the chance to see a good Yang-style swordsman in action.
- Any applications should look balanced, connected, and realistic in the sense that they might work, at the very least, against a committed attacker and not just as a two-person dance. As I suggested earlier, constant blocking and clashing of weapons is a sign that the level of skill being shown is rudimentary at best. This kind of sword fencing emphasizes footwork, positioning, and deflections. The emphasis is on sensitivity and using "sticky" circling methods as a way of learning how to suddenly disengage your weapon while cutting the hand or wrist of the opponent's hand to (somewhat literally) disarm him. Conversely, you also need to develop skill at countercircling to avoid those wrist cuts!
- A jian is never allowed to move directly above the crown of the wielder's head for a variety of reasons that are practical (it might be struck down into you so

that you cut yourself with the edge facing your body) and esoteric (you wouldn't want to sever your connection with the Yang energy of Heaven entering the baihui point on the top of your head). I should also add that some styles will use sword techniques that make it look superficially as if the sword has gone over the head. If you examine the posture carefully, however, you will see that the wielder has actually swung his arm over his head and not the edged part of the blade. Of course, to the casual observer there isn't much apparent difference, but the wielder is less likely to cut or hit himself with the sword in this way. Such moves are usually defensive and meant to stop an attack from the rear, or sometimes to launch an attack from an unusual angle of entry.

- The left hand is usually held in the "sword-amulet" (jianque) position—first two fingers straight, thumb, ring, and little fingers making a loose circle. This is symbolic of the magic sword used by Buddhist/Daoist priests to slay evil spirits. This hand position was also meant in part to provide physical balance of feel in the empty hand to match the hand holding the sword. It was also meant to circulate the qi in the empty hand to balance the internal energy flow, and it could be used under certain martial circumstances to strike vulnerable parts of the attacker's anatomy. After all, it is the person holding the sword who is dangerous, and not just the sword itself.
- A few modern teachers also suggest that it really represented a way of carrying a small knife in the other hand that could be "flicked-out" for a surprise attack. Considering the traditional Chinese love for small concealable weapons, this is hardly an unreasonable suggestion. By the way, Dr. Yang Jwing-ming has written an excellent and interesting book—*Ancient Chinese*

Weapons—that, I believe, is still in print and available through his Web site, www.ymaasa.co.za.

Practical Considerations for Sword Training

I would recommend that you start your training with a wooden sword, as the weight is less likely to strain your wrist or challenge your shoulders in the way that a metal weapon can. I should add, though, that some instructors would argue that you should always train with metal weapons to get some sense of the proper weight and balance, and to learn to treat what you are doing with respect. As even a blunt metal weapon can cause serious injuries, using such encourages most students to be precise and serious about their training.

My own feeling is that it is best to practice applications only with wooden weapons at first. This is not just for safety, but also to minimize the strain in your wrists and arms from the extra weight of the weapon itself. Practice with metal weapons can be reserved for solo and two-person forms. It also doesn't hurt to wear safety glasses, helmets, and protective gear on your hands, forearms, and elbows, as these are prime targets for many techniques. You can also improvise more complete protective suits from hockey, lacrosse,and BMX bicycling gear and (as a bonus) you'll get to feel like you are an extra in *The Road Warrior.*

It is also important to train with blunt metal weapons to see the difference weight and feel can bring to your techniques. I don't like using padded plastic weapons, as has become popular in recent years at competitive events, because they are so light that they move too quickly. Being hit with one doesn't hurt much, so defensive tactics don't tend to be learned and instead we are left with a game of tag.

Being able to understand how the jian works at a variety of ranges and against a variety of weapons or opponents is what really matters and, in the end, it's how much and how well you learn this that brings the beginnings of true skill. I have also read and been told by more than one instructor that the intensive study of the sword is an excellent way to both health and enlightenment in the long run.

Certainly, the sword has been imbued with a spiritual quality in many societies—both Western and Oriental. I'm sure Sigmund Freud would have something to say about the significance of swords to men, but then again, he seems to have been more than a little obsessed with the penis himself!

I went through a long period of time in which I had little interest in traditional weapons training of any kind, but now I derive a great deal of satisfaction from the sword form(s) that I practice and with the short staff forms that I learned from Erle Montaigue.

FINAL WORDS ON WEAPONS TRAINING

In taiji terms, it is important to have fundamental martial skills in whatever version of that art you are studying before moving on to the traditional weapons, particularly the jian, as it demands so much unity in the movements of the wrist, waist, and footwork. Do I also have to repeat that it is important to have a teacher who understands at least basic usage of the weapon, as opposed to a teacher who focuses on solo forms?

Even a marginal understanding of combative function will make your forms as challenging and rewarding as they are fun. However, true skill with any traditional weapon comes from practicing and experimenting (and a few bruises and splinters from using wooden copies of the weapons).

Any such practice needs lots of space for indoor practice—an important consideration as with any of the more traditional forms. There's literally no point in learning the weapon if you can't practice it for lack of training space—remember winter? Practicing in a park is one option, but North America isn't China and pedestrians aren't used to the sight of flailing swords and sabers the way they are in Shanghai or Beijing.

If you are planning to practice in the park or your back yard, you'll need a fair bit of privacy. One of my former senior students had the police arrive to question him more than once while practicing in parks when someone reported that "some crazy guy is waving a sword in the park."

UNITING THE FIVE PILLARS

Very few people will be attracted to all the martial training aspects as I have described in the past pages, while even fewer will develop any real skill at all of those aspects of the "hard" side of the Yang style. Fewer still will have the inclination and the aptitude to exceed such intermediate levels of martial understanding.

At this stage, you have actually started to go beyond individual techniques and formal two-person training to learn to be a little more spontaneous in your martial reactions, and to do so while under more pressure from those you train with as well as your teacher.

In this regard, it is essential to remember that the Chinese meaning of san sau is really more akin to "free hands," with the implication of free-for-all training or self-defense.

Unarmed Self-Defense

At this level, you must learn how to close the distance between yourself and the other person automatically and be able to neutralize and yield as you counterattack, while having some idea of how to deal with a variety of styles of attack (a puncher, a grabber, a thrower, or any combination thereof).

Having this kind of training environment is difficult, as it requires one-on-one coaching or relatively small groups and a willingness by both the attacker as well as the defender to escalate the violence only as much as each participant can manage at a given time in their development. In other words, there has to be a spirit of cooperation, even though this kind of training is not done cooperatively!

In the long run, any real combative skill you develop will result from internalizing the principles of taiji and a relatively few techniques, as opposed to learning many applications on a superficial level. This small arsenal can eventually become internal (or instinctive, or subconscious, or a conditioned reflex—call it what you like). One way to do this is to select a few postures from the solo form(s) that you do particularly well or like the most and practice them endlessly, both on your own and with a partner.

Try to pick methods that cover attacks from the most common angles and from both the right and left sides. If you can eventually make them work while being attacked with some speed and power, then you're on the right track. These postures can be done a variety of ways depending on how skillful you and your partner are and whether you have the skill to counter whatever he or she may throw at you as a follow-up method.

It is important to practice doing the applications in a variety of ways: practicing striking or kicking the air at a variety of paces, hitting a focus mitt held by a partner or a heavy bag so that you learn how important it is to have the right shape to your wrist and fist or palm when striking, and how to kick something without knocking yourself over in the process.

Remember that there is really no one ideal application for each posture (although some experts would no doubt argue with this). I believe that each posture has one or more interpretations as a defense against either being struck or grabbed, but each will also have countless variations depending on the skills and strengths of the practitioner as well as the angle and complexity of attack.

As I said before, in the end, you learn techniques to transcend them. Otherwise, you remain merely a competent technician rather than someone who can face the unexpected with any hope of surviving it.

In attempting to reduce the necessary factors to a manageable number, you could say that there are four essential unarmed self-defense skills:

- Dominating the initial contact: When you touch the opponent with your arm or hand while deflecting/neutralizing the attacking limb, you use that contact to control or "rub" the limb so as to distract him (even momentarily) as well as hopefully upsetting his balance. Doing this can also provide an opportunity to lock up one or more joints, strike with the other hand, or throw or trip.
- Stealing the timing: When the opponent doesn't want to take the initiative, you must either feint an attack or extend a hand, inviting the opponent to make contact with you. Once this contact is made you can use the "bridge" you have created to attack. This tactic can be particularly useful against those who have mistaken the forest for the trees through martial training that has conditioned them to get too close even when this is counterproductive. This leads us to the third point.
- Breaking contact, if necessary: If the opponent has skill and successfully grabs your arm(s) or body, you must have the skill to break that contact by withdrawing while counterattacking to distract him from pressing his advantage or from reestablishing effective martial contact.

- Sticking and striking/throwing/controlling until it is not necessary to continue to do so: If your opponent tries to break the bridge you have created, you must follow his actions to maintain contact with one hand or a part of your body while you continue to attack until it is no longer necessary to do so.

There are many reasons to do taiji. Understanding the principles is important, as is practicing in a safe and controlled manner, but it's also easy to close your eyes to how effective what you are doing might be if your life depended on it. For the few that have the interest, there are many training methods that can teach the basics of self-defense skills done with relaxation and the requisite whole-body mechanics, but they require a willingness to sweat and suffer a few bruises, both to the body and the ego. They also require patience.

It bears repeating that practicing the solo aspects of taiji won't bring significant self-defense skills unless you learn and practice that side of the art with a competent teacher for several years. You can't learn fighting by osmosis if all you ever do is meditate and do a slow form.

Conversely, those students who do those things regularly may find that they learn the self-defense stuff more efficiently than those who approach the martial side of taiji without an inner peace and some kind of understanding of the basic concepts of how to move in a determined and connected manner that is true to the taiji legacy.

Self-Defense Against Knives and Clubs

A famous man (no, whoops, that was me) once wrote in an article for a British police magazine (Police Review, Vol. 95, November 13, 1987) that the key to defending against a knife was to remember your mother's good advice when you were little and she caught you fiddling with the kitchen cutlery: "Don't play with that, you'll get cut!"

Mom was right. In fact, the hardest aspect of defending against a knife is getting used to the idea that you can't be overly concerned about avoiding all cuts, as you will probably have to sacrifice a piece of yourself to get the knife wielder. I don't often go into the specifics of defending against such weapons with my students because I do feel that it is relatively useless to learn knife or club defenses until you already have considerable physical skill in all the other unarmed self-defense basics.

By the way, I should acknowledge that some very competent martial artists argue the exact opposite, that you should learn how to fight with and defend against such weapons first in your training, then translate those skills to unarmed tactics—but we are talking about Yang taiji.

In recent years, a variety of experts have produced a huge volume of videos and DVDs on defending against knives. They run the gamut from the laughable to those like Erle Montaigue's, which give pragmatic advice on this topic.

To summarize Erle's approach to knife defense (and I do recommend his videos on the topic):

- Evade (get out of the way)
- Bump (strike the arm holding the knife in the joints, or where the nerve endings come close to the surface, away from you both to cause pain and, hopefully, knock the weapon loose from the attacker's grip)
- Attack vital points (eyes and throat)

In unarmed self-defense you might be able to accept a blow to the torso in order to strike a more vital area on your opponent, but this cannot work against someone armed with a knife. Even a small, accidental cut to an artery can cause you to go into shock or bleed to death in a very short period of time. The point of a knife is often so small and sharp that only a relatively light amount of force is required for deep penetration, which can lead to severe infection and death, even with medical attention.

Similarly, an experienced knife fighter will expect you to block or grab the hand holding the weapon and many are prepared to fold at the elbow to continue attacking you despite your grip. Many are strong enough to pull and twist the blade back to sever your fingers as you try to hold their attacking arm.

More importantly, most techniques in unarmed martial arts require great skill to have any success of working, but the attacker's knife hand will often move very quickly and erratically. Very little body force is necessary to inflict deep cuts with a sharp knife and it takes relatively little practice to be able to attack successfully with a knife when you don't care how badly the target is hurt, especially compared to how long it takes to learn how to defend against such attacks.

I am a rather mild-mannered martial artist in most ways, but in an attempt to make my teenage sons understand how I viewed the idea of carrying knives, as teenagers sometimes are tempted to do, I told them that I would, with great regret afterward, have to try to kill anyone like them that pulled a knife on me on the street. You can't take chances and even a skinny 13-year-old can cut you enough to kill you if you don't get immediate medical aid. I also pointed out that pulling a knife is stupid unless you are sure that you can hang on to it so that it doesn't end up being used against you. I suspect that it was the latter argument that had the most impact on their adolescent minds.

It is essential to remember in all aspects of such training that you must be as concerned with the person holding the weapon as with the weapon itself. For example, the sudden appearance of such a weapon in an attacker's hand may prove distracting to the point where the attacker can stab or slash you when you freeze in fear, or he can kick or strike you with his free hand while you stare at the knife or club and then use his weapon at his leisure.

Being clubbed is similar to being attacked with a knife, although it is marginally easier to defend against someone using a blunt impact weapon if you have any skill at all. A broken arm can be survived if it means you take out the attacker and you were only faced by one aggressor, but a slashed throat earned while crippling your attacker is a very poor trade indeed! In addition, you may be able roll with the impact of a blunt weapon if it is hitting a muscular portion of your body in order to counterattack, but this is still risky business.

As with any aspect of self-defense, you need to have excellent martial skills and practice both with and against the common ways of swinging and wielding a knife or club to have any hope of being able to do so on the street.

It is important to remember that you have to learn how to handle these weapons offensively with some ability to learn how to adequately defend against them. As I mentioned before, this holds true of unarmed techniques as well. You can't learn to defend yourself properly if you have no idea of how to attack in a realistic and effective manner, and vice-versa.

FINAL THOUGHTS ON SELF-DEFENSE IN GENERAL

In the end, it is not possible to learn self-defense or combative skills that might work against a skilled or determined attacker without controlled contact and some form of spontaneous unrehearsed attacks, albeit in a controlled manner, with or without body armor.

Having this kind of training environment is difficult, as it requires one-on-one coaching or very small groups and a willingness by both the attacker and the defender to escalate the "violence" only as much as each participant can manage at a given time in their development. In other words, there has to be a spirit of cooperation, even though this kind of training is not done cooperatively.

As with all training, it is important to practice with a variety of partners. Tall people can learn to use the reach of their long arms even more effectively, short people can learn to use a low center of gravity to "get inside" a taller person's reach, heavy people can learn to use their mass even more effectively, slim people can learn to use their flexibility to even greater effect, etc.

NO martial training can guarantee that you will be able to successfully defend yourself against any aggressor. No one knows how they will react in a particular type of situation unless they have been exposed to that kind of situation. It's called experience and, as the saying goes, it makes you or it breaks you. There's also paranoia and spending a lot of time analyzing whether strangers will be dangerous when you should be focusing on being a better, more peaceful person yourself.

Fortunately, few of us will ever have to use our martial skills for anything more demanding than friendly practice. However, such training should give you a "fighting chance" and, while some aggressors may lose "heart" for a fight if you hit them first and well and repeatedly if you are forced into that kind of situation, some aggressors will just smile a little and get even meaner, even if you hit them well.

In the end, training is not the same as fighting and Murphy's Law ("If something can go wrong it will!") always applies—as does the old adage, "Keep it simple, stupid!"

In light of scientific research, not to mention common sense, it would seem obvious that the traditional styles (e.g., Yang family and Chen) or those that have fast or slow/fast forms (e.g., Tung family fast set) would be of the greatest use in terms of both cardiovascular health as well as maximizing stress reduction. In fact, a vigorous workout is more effective in stimulating the body to produce endorphins, those chemicals that promote a sense of well-being.

In addition, such vigorous workouts raise the body temperature, which triggers certain chemical changes in the brain that help ease anxiety (hot showers and saunas have much the same effect). Of course, this does not mean that you should abandon doing the long, slow form—only that you should supplement its practice with a fast form or some type of cardiovascular training.

There are lots of reasons to do taijiquan or any martial art beyond just being a capable fighter. On the other hand, most practitioners never go much beyond focusing on whatever aspect of the training that they are good at or that interests them the most.

I think that the study of something like Yang style taijiquan should bring competent self-defense skills as well as improve your health and, in the long run, make you a more mature human being.

ENDNOTE

1. Hair-shirt training is even harder to find than iron shirt training, as it is an old "hidden system" in Christianity for teaching humility and reflecting on your sins. As you can imagine, almost no one practices this anymore.

Chapter 6
Controversial Issues

Many beginners come to their first taijiquan class thinking that there is only one form of taiji out there instead of countless variations—both good and bad. However, even more experienced students may be astounded to learn that there there is as much difference of opinion about almost ANY taiji-related issue as there are people talking about that subject.

Aside from attending workshops and competitions, one way to experience this is to visit any of the taiji or internal arts Internet discussion boards, although the level of sophistication in the discussions is often on a par with that generated in a redneck bar on Saturday night or a schoolyard full of adolescents.

In this chapter, I would like to touch on the most important of the contentious topics that are frequently raised when experienced practitioners get together to discuss the issues dear to their heart in a friendly, and sometimes not so friendly, manner.

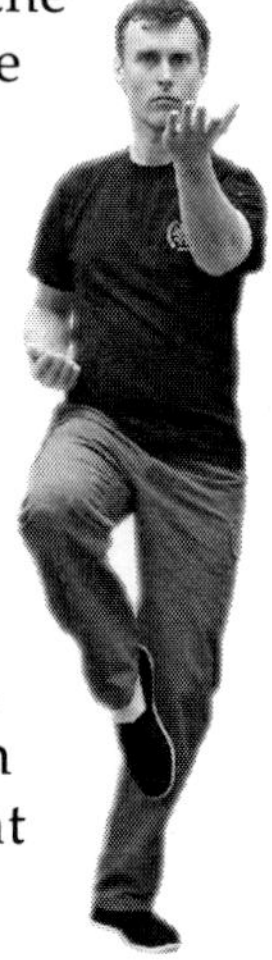

INSTRUCTIONAL ISSUES

Will the Real Yang Style Please Step Forward?

A cynic who has done some research and gone to the bother of comparing modern approaches to the Yang style might think that even the family versions have changed a great deal since the mid-19th century. One group of experts says or implies that the modern versions are concise and stripped-down in relation to the needless complexity and difficulty of the original versions of the Yang style. The opposing camp says or implies that the modern versions are debased and simplistic versions of the originals. While older is not necessarily better, it remains true that many of the variations developed since the Second World War may be suitable for beginners, but don't have enough depth to sustain those who want to develop more than a superficial understanding of the art.

When you compare the long solo forms and martial training methods taught by a few instructors to the majority of interpretations of the Yang style that you commonly meet, it should be obvious to the discriminating that something has gone rather wrong in the process of transmission.

Sometimes this is deliberate, as when an expert changes a form to conceal its essence from outsiders, but more often the problem lies in the quality of the intermediaries between the student and the originator of a style. In general, the fewer people involved, the less chance there is of serious errors being introduced. Think of it this way: Would you rather own the master recording of a symphony done with professional equipment or the copy you made from a bootleg somebody else made with amateur recording equipment?

Even with the highest skill and best intentions, some changes occur every time a form is learned by a new teacher and subsequently passed on to his or her disciples for further transmission. Yang taijiquan, in particular, is burdened with endless bad copies of bad copies.

A student learns briefly from a reputable instructor and then, without the teacher's blessing, goes off to teach students who do the same after an equally inadequate apprenticeship. The original form becomes riddled with errors or changes are made for all the wrong reasons. In addition, many of the current generation of teachers have never studied a martial art of any kind, much less had valid training in a complete curriculum of the combative side of taiji.

To make it even harder to find quality instruction, many of those who have real skill stop teaching because of age or health issues, or just because good students are rare compared to the numbers of elderly, overweight, middle-class, and sedentary recruits to the Yang style.

Leaving aside for the moment the tricky issue of deciphering lineage and deciding who has the real goods from a technical and historical perspective, a large part of the historical difference between traditional and modern taiji is the relationship between the student and the teacher. In traditional schools, the master was very selective of his students. He usually had only a few and these had been recommended by a close friend, family member, or other martial arts master. The prospective student had to undergo a formal ceremony of swearing allegiance to his new master.

After years of training and proving himself, he then might become an "inner door disciple" (tude) and be shown the secrets of the art. At this level, he was also expected to treat his teacher literally like an adoptive father and extend the requisite financial and personal support due to the head of the family in China. Eventually, the best of this elite was then selected and groomed in the last remaining secret training techniques to be the next lineage holder after the master retired or died. This kind of intensive and long-term, one-on-one coaching tended to produce quality practitioners—but not many of them. And, occasionally, the heir-apparent would die prematurely and unexpectedly, with disastrous results for the style in question.

Of course, I have also heard it suggested in modern times that being a lineage holder is not always indicative that the best person has been selected to carry on the tradition. Sometimes the selection is based on family politics or simply used as a way of rewarding whoever is willing to look after the old master in his declining years.

In a modern setting, a taiji teacher is often willing to accept anyone who has an apparent interest in learning the art. In the better examples of this approach, the teacher will be teaching as a hobby, not as a means of earning a living, and restricts his teaching to small numbers of students whom he does his best to teach to the best of their learning abilities.

By contrast, in the more commercial schools, the teaching may still have quality but be geared to those few natural athletes and fighters and not to the needs of the majority of the students. This dumbing-down process can degenerate even further if the teacher's main criteria for admittance becomes a new student's willingness to pay the required fees.

In such an environment, class size is frequently excessive and geared to making as much profit as possible for as little real effort as possible on the part of the teacher or school owner. In such cases, the martial training is usually modified to retain students and minimize the chance of litigation over accidental injuries.

Getting back to the issue of lineage, it is usually the skill of each individual teacher of that style as well as the skill of each individual student that will decide how valid the material is for those who study it, though you wouldn't know this from the large numbers of modern teachers whom you meet who cover their walls with certificates and flow charts of their lineage.

It should be obvious to those with common sense that having a famous father or famous teacher won't guarantee that you have any aspect of that person's skill or genius, but common sense is often ignored in the modern expressions of the internal martial arts. Longer history may make a system more durable and adaptable, but it is just as likely to make it a museum piece only suitable for those obsessed with the past.

Though I know that many of my conservative colleagues will disagree, I don't think that there is any way around the necessity for change in even the best forms and training methods. Otherwise, the art becomes, as I said, a museum piece with relevance only to those obsessed with the past. Some of the changes one can see in the decent modern versions of the Yang style have been for the better.

For example, the teachers who have studied sports science or medicine in university or college have realized that these disciplines understand human physiology and how to train safely and effectively much better than the old masters. Similarly, the traditional way of teaching in which information was given out sparingly and questions were discouraged unless you were one of the teacher's chosen elite has been replaced in better schools with a spirit of inquiry that would be alien to an old-style master.

However, too much or needless change can also cause problems and I do think that it is important to leave a legacy for future Yang generations that has continuity with the past. For this reason, as well as in tribute to the inherent genius of those who created them, I don't think that the solo forms of the family styles should be consciously changed, but rather should be passed on with all the accuracy that each teacher is capable of.

For these reasons, I have been creative only in very in small ways in my own teaching as my skills have evolved, but I have not consciously changed the traditional forms as I have learned them from those who taught me. My only problem with creativity is when some teachers refuse to acknowledge their work and attribute their inventions to mysterious Chinese gentlemen who happened to live next door to them. This is suspicious even in the Orient and was unlikely in North America or Europe until fairly recently.

However, life has a habit of producing exceptions to the rule at every turn and it has been my experience that you shouldn't also get overly cynical about the possibilities of a white expert having met or learned from a qualified Chinese teacher in even the strangest locales. The tide of Chinese immigration is rising in the last two decades, and many intermediate and high level masters have moved to the West. For example, Yang Jun, who as Yang Zhen Duo's grandson is being groomed to be the next head of the Yang family, is now an American citizen. The head of another version of the Yang family, Fu Shen Yuan, is now a citizen of Australia.

It is also important to remember that modern experts are often bringing aspects of their other fighting or healing experience to whatever taiji forms and methods that they teach, so that the information is rarely from a pure taiji or pure Yang perspective. This is unavoidable and, in the early days, those attracted to taijiquan were often older men with a lifetime of martial training under their belts.

In the same way that a prestigious lineage cannot guarantee that a particular teacher will automatically be talented, just because a a taijiquan organization is large and has a famous teacher as a figurehead will not guarantee competent instruction in any of the member schools you might come into contact with in your particular area. Also, you should never assume that a teacher is less competent on any level because he is not Chinese or because you have never heard of him or his teachers (and vice versa).

Some taijiquan organizations are sometimes shams in the sense that they exist only on paper, or the members have bought a certificate by sending in the required membership fee or visiting a famous master for a week or two in China. There are always otherwise reputable teachers in China who are not in the least bit shy in handing out certificates to any foreigner who comes with enough money and an introduction from someone they know overseas.

In the end, both the modern and traditional approaches have their respective merits and both approaches are also easy to overdo—the traditionalists become obsessed with historical accuracy over practicality, while the nontraditionalists can be too quick to throw out whatever does not appeal to them and change forms and methods for all the wrong reasons.

Finding the original solo form or the original push-hands method of the Yang style is highly unlikely, but finding a good teacher with access to one of the better inheritances and variations of this discipline is both possible and crucial if you want to have some hope of developing even a pale reflection of the original art.

Which is Better: Group or Private Instruction?

Having found a suitable instructor, some people will choose private instruction because that teacher does not offer group classes that meet their needs in terms of day-to-day scheduling and family or work responsibilities. Similarly, some students might prefer private instruction but simply not have the financial freedom to pursue these as opposed to the normally substantially cheaper option of group classes. Fortunately, each learning environment brings its own unique challenges and joys.

Some people hate practicing with others or being watched while they learn new things, others love showing off, while some couldn't care less if they are being either watched or ignored as they train. Some find it distracting to their ability to pay attention to what they are either being taught or are trying to practice if they have people moving around them, while others need to be able to watch those around them while practicing to have any hope of keeping up with the group effort.

In the end, there are a number of issues, besides those just mentioned, to be considered when deciding whether group or private instruction is best for you.

Group Instruction

Except for that small minority of people who can only tolerate their own company, human beings are very much social animals. So, it shouldn't be a surprise that group practice is the most common vehicle for studying taijiquan. A common benefit of group practice in relation to the long, slow form in particular is that it usually ensures that those moving too quickly must slow their pace, while those who are slow by reason of pausing awkwardly, here and there, are encouraged to accelerate their movements as appropriate in order to keep pace.

Much in the same way that clock pendulums in one room will eventually move in a synchronized manner, even if initially swinging at different tempos, humans tend both consciously and subconsciously to do the same. This phenomena—particularly in qigong and slow form training—can also create a cumulative energetic benefit for the individuals who make up the group practicing together. This is known as jenqi to the Chinese and is said to be the energy created by a group of people acting harmoniously together. A Westerner might think of it in terms of a "positive vibe" being created by and for the group.

Of course, it's difficult to analyze where the psychology of group dynamics begins and where jenqi leaves off, but it remains true that a group of committed practitioners doing qigong and solo form together can generate an atmosphere conducive to smiles, if nothing else, while practicing together. Good instructors encourage this to assist in the healing aspects the training. Unfortunately, unscrupulous instructors can also use it as a forum to influence their students to do things that they might not otherwise want to do when on their own.

It is an interesting phenomenon from the teacher's perspective that many students with months, sometimes years of experience are able to do a solo form semicompetently while in a group, but cannot do so when training on their own. This is sometimes due to memory-loss problems in older students, sometimes due to lack of regular personal practice, and sometimes due to any of a variety of fairly common learning disabilities.

The only real downside, from a teacher's perspective, to group classes is that some people focus on the social aspects and spend too much time talking with each other or trying to find their next sexual partner. Many taiji environments also seem to encourage drinking tea and eating fancy sandwiches and pastries more than the actual training. Pleasant though such activities may be, it tends to waste precious class time that could be devoted to learning new skills and reinforcing old ones.

It should be obvious that group classes are also essential for martial training. Variety in training partners is essential for long-term skill building. In particular, the more experienced student can only benefit from training with a variety of body types and skill levels and not just one person—even if that one person is the instructor. Group classes become essential for those who started with private sessions and want to maximize their martial training.

Private Instruction

Private instruction certainly is preferable in many ways as a way of learning simply because the student has all of the attention of the teacher and can benefit from that in the sense of getting immediate feedback on what is being learned, practiced, or asked. Many people will feel less shy about asking questions in a private session.

On the other hand, questions—and answering them—are often a waste of time in a group session, as many who are attracted to taiji in North America are overly intellectual in their approach and sometimes are trying to show how much they already know with their questions instead of trying to learn. Even if that is not the case, those who didn't ask the question will rarely listen enough to benefit from whatever advice you may hand out on the issue.

In addition, whether in a private or group class, if the person asking the question is a relative beginner, he or she may just not have enough experience to make an answer relevant to what they are practicing.

Questions only start to be stupid when the person asking them doesn't listen to the answers. By the way, this is not the same thing as failing to understand, in the sense that a good teacher will not necessarily expect you to completely understand any answer the first time.

Of course, a one-on-one classroom relationship can be counterproductive if the instructor is unscrupulous and tries to dominate the student emotionally to abuse them either financially or sexually.

On a more positive note, private instruction in martial techniques and skills is extremely useful for experienced students, as this kind of coaching from someone who has "the touch" and does not rely on crude force for martial purposes can really bring new insights to the student. In addition, many students will be able to practice better with the teacher than with their peers for a variety of reasons, including having more respect for the teacher because of his or her position of authority. They will also be able to refrain from being overly competitive with the teacher, unlike the dual of egos that often overtakes two students of a similar level of skill who train together.

Particularly when the student is experienced, motivated, and has some aptitude, private martial classes can bring progress that might otherwise take much longer in a group training format. On the other hand, private martial instruction for beginners is less useful because the student will not yet have the basic skills or experience to appreciate the subtle differences between what the teacher and he or she can do.

Final Thoughts on Group vs. Private Instruction

The decision to embrace or avoid group classes is often driven more by the personality of the would-be student than by any other factor related to getting the best possible instruction. In my experience as a teacher, I have found that a significant proportion of those seeking private instruction do so for the wrong reasons, be it a fear of looking awkward in front of other students, or a desire to have the instructor all to themselves.

Neither attitude is necessarily fatal to a student's progress as long as that student can outgrow such attitudes as he or she progresses in his or her studies. Sadly, many do not. Perhaps in the end the ideal for both teacher and student alike lies in small group classes so that a sense of family can develop, and so that a variety of training partners are available without sacrificing the benefits of having detailed feedback and instruction.

Of course, this kind of class precludes the teacher being able to afford a large commercial school setting, which requires a large number of students to pay the bills, much less make a profit. In the end, the search for *quality* instruction often seems to take us back to the time-honored tradition of teaching out of one's home or in a public park.

IS HAVING FAITH A DOUBLE-EDGED SWORD?

Robert Smith wrote in his groundbreaking book, *T'ai Chi,* (Charles E. Tuttle Co., Vermont, 1967) of having asked his teacher and co-author, the famous Cheng Man Ching, why none of the latter's students approached his skill levels. Cheng replied that it was due to a lack of faith on their part. Such a simple answer is sometimes difficult to accept for those modern students whose minds are either a little too active or who interpret everything in purely mechanical terms.

For more experienced students, faith can make almost anything possible once the physical skills start to fall into place. As in most aspects of life, it is important to keep an open mind, and analyzing taijiquan is of less value than knowing if doing any aspect of it in a competent manner will make you a healthier and more skillful person on many levels.

Seen this way, the self-healing side of taiji is less a question of trying to master or control yourself or your internal energy and more a question of setting realistic goals and working toward them. Perhaps the process of finding faith both in one's self and in one's teacher(s) is similar to the leap of faith that a more experienced taiji practitioner must undergo to transcend the limitations of practicing the forms and methods on a technical basis.

If one of my students doesn't believe that he or she can do a successful technique against whatever I direct his or her way in the martial training, it would hardly be surprising if they didn't do as well as they should be able to in objective terms. On the other hand, misplaced faith is bad enough when limited to incompetently taught solo practice. It is even worse when the instructor claims to teach martial techniques that, in reality, would only work on a student who is subconsciously cooperating with the teacher.

For example, if I tell my students that I will be able to attract them toward me with the qi I can project from my hand, by hovering that hand close to their chests, it will work with a significant proportion of them. If I then explain that it's not really the power of my internal energy but just their subconscious cooperation (i.e., autosuggestion) to their teacher moving his hand smoothly toward and then away from them, it will *still* work on a significant proportion of the students—even though their intellectual minds knows that it's a trick.

One of my former teachers used to tell the story of the time he was teaching a qigong workshop to a group of strangers. As is often the case, there was one loud, disruptive person in the group who kept interrupting and asking stupid questions. At a break time, he told my teacher that he was experiencing stomach aches and cramping and went on and on about it even though everyone was trying to leave to go for lunch.

In a moment of irritation, my former teacher made up a simple qigong exercise out of thin air. He told the complainer to go stand in the corner for 20 minutes while doing the nonsense exercise and he would feel better afterward. The loudmouth did what was suggested and later reported that he felt much better after the "miraculous" qigong.

The power of the mind when it believes that healing is taking place should not be underestimated, and there seems to be limitless numbers of such people attracted to both qigong and Yang-style taiji in particular (not to mention to the television evangelists). Sadly, there is a great deal of this misuse of faith in the modern taijiquan universe and I will go into more detail on that in the section on separating martial fact from fantasy.

Certainly, a student must have faith in himself or herself on many levels, as well as faith in the teacher and in the material being learned. It is a shame that so many North American students of taijiquan choose to immerse themselves rather too wholeheartedly in their fantasies rather than acknowledging that the Orient does not have a monopoly on wisdom, any more than does the West. Similarly, placing your teacher on a pedestal is probably not too healthy for either the student or the subject of his or her infatuation.

ARE TAIJI COMPETITIONS AND WORKSHOPS USEFUL?

Once you have developed some real skill and experience, I would strongly suggest that you do as many workshops and attend as many taiji events as you can afford in terms of your finances and time constraints. It's very difficult to continue to evolve as a practitioner the longer you practice. A stunted growth is more likely to occur when you, consciously or subconsciously, compare yourself to your immediate classmates and think, "I'm far ahead of these people."

It is easy to forget that there is a much larger taiji world outside the boundaries of your immediate school. Skill as a practitioner and teacher is always relative in the sense that you may be more skilled and experienced than your classmates, but not of those with a comparable amount of experience in another teacher's taiji class or in the general martial arts community.

Similarly, as a teacher, you may have more skill than your students, but much less than anyone with comparable years of experience who is teaching elsewhere in your geographical area. A few taiji experts, either because of their skill or good publicity, do become famous enough to give workshops or teach and demonstrate at the major competitive events.

So it will also probably be true that, if you are practicing or teaching on a recreational level, your abilities will probably be less than those of the few professional taijiquan teachers whom you may meet through such venues. Again, the unfortunate tendency is for even these few paragons to compare themselves to the local teachers of taiji and martial arts and think, consciously or subconsciously, "I'm far ahead of them."

It bears repeating that it is essential for any level of practitioner to make the effort to compare what he or she is doing with what is going on in the larger taiji world. It is easy to remain a "big fish in a small pond." You have to make some effort to compare notes with the fish in the ocean if you are serious about your interest in becoming competent.

Competitions

Such events allow you to see or experience a variety of experts and "would-be" experts performing or teaching aspects of their arts. You can gain insights by hearing the same topics discussed in a new way, learn forms and training methods that are not covered by your regular teacher, practice push-hands and a variety of training methods with a variety of people, and perhaps make new friends as well as engage in taiji-related discussions to your heart's content. I've met some wonderful people (and also a few who are anything but!) by traveling to such events and by doing workshops with a variety of instructors.

However, I don't think that the serious taijiquan student should routinely enter into the competitive side of taiji. What do winning medals, wearing fancy silk uniforms, and participating in pushing contests that usually look like incompetent judo have to do with any of the traditional aspects of taiji? In particular, the martial sport skills that are necessary to win contests are often inconsistent with realistic self-defense skills in that they are too restricted in terms of allowed techniques and footwork. The reason given for this is usually the safety of the participants, even though full-contact fighting is permitted in boxing and Mixed Martial Arts (MMA) competitions.

The participants in the latter venues normally survive the hard knocks and minor injuries that result from this kind of competition. Why should taiji be approached differently for those who want to compete in this way? Surely experienced players can strike with controlled intensity that limits the potential for injury while allowing the judges to see the potential effectiveness of such tactics. Similarly, such strikes can be evaded, absorbed, or neutralized as well as any other and grappling can be executed to the level of controlling the opponent without causing serious injury.

Certainly the present lackluster state of taiji competition push-hands in terms of martial realism does much to aid the general perception outside the art that it is being done in an ineffective manner compared to disciplines and martial sports like Brazilian jiu-jitsu, Thai boxing, la boxe Francaise, much less Western boxing or MMA. Of course, one could also add with some justification that the philosophical ideas often ascribed to taijiquan go against the idea of competing for ultimately meaningless prizes and honors. While the ethics of nonviolence and defensive force may well be fairly recent additions to taijiquan, training to fight competitively does go against the noble idea of the art being a means of self-defense and not just a means of imposing one's superiority over others. There is more to life than fighting. A good variation of taijiquan should provide both self-healing and martial training in equal measure, although having been young once myself, I understand why young men compete with one another.

Having said all of this, I also think that a serious student of taijiquan should have the experience of demonstrating form in front of a large audience or participating in a solo form competition, at least once during his or her taiji career. The extra practice and attention to detail in your physical conditioning and overall practice before doing such is like eating your grandmother's chicken soup when you have the flu—it can't hurt and may help.

It's equally true that many of those watching in an audience of that kind wouldn't know indifferent or quality taijiquan from bad, but that shouldn't stop you from doing your best while all those eyes are on you.

Workshops

It has been suggested that middle-class North Americans in particular are "workshop junkies" and, while this is hardly a fair generalization, it is also true that workshops are often a waste of time and money in terms of a student being able to take away much of benefit. I was discussing this issue with a colleague and we agreed that only the best and the worst practitioners attended a lot of workshops. (Hopefully, he and I both fall in the first category.)

One of the most obvious effects of the growth in popularity of taijiquan has been the proliferation of workshops in most aspects of the art. Most cities of any size will have or host such events on a semiregular basis at the very least. One that is of particular interest to those living in the United States is the *A Taste of China* summer seminars, workshops, and demonstrations held annually in the state of Virginia (www.atoctaijiquan.com). This week-long event attracts teachers and students of all the internal and external Chinese martial disciplines and has been doing so for more than 20 years.

Keep in mind that the better workshops or training camps will be very difficult to afford more than once or twice a year and that attending a session in which you are one of 50–75 attendees will mean that you may come away with very little in terms of long-lasting information. Too many seem content to take endless workshops just to get a photo with or a few memories of the guest instructor, not to mention the certificates and T-shirts that are handed out or sold at such events.

To get the most out of attending workshops, try to find a good teacher who regularly travels to an area to which you can realistically afford to travel at least once a year, and attend such sessions with a training partner from your area with whom you can practice regularly until the next workshop.

It is a strange phenomenon, in my experience, that many practitioners who could easily afford to do so will not even bother to attend workshops that are conveniently held in their taiji club or city—much less travel anywhere outside their home base to do so. This is sometimes due to lack of time and financial resources, sometimes to laziness, and sometimes to the kind of blind loyalty that drives some students to think that it is disrespectful to their teacher to look elsewhere for inspiration. Conversely, a good teacher will want you someday to be as skillful as he or she is; an excellent teacher will want you to surpass his or her achievements.

SHOULD YOU JOIN A TAIJI OR MARTIAL ASSOCIATION?

No matter what your level of experience, there's a great deal of value to being part of a taiji or martial arts association. Unfortunately, there's also a great deal to be said for not wasting your time with them. Over the years, I have been in several such associations and, depending on who you study with, you sometimes won't have a choice as to whether you join or participate in a particular association. Involuntary "volunteering" at the behest of a Chinese teacher is a common enough expectation in the traditional martial arts world to which taijiquan belongs.

The Good Aspects

As with workshops, being part of a larger body of like-minded individuals can be very eye-opening in the sense of allowing you to see the art expressed in a variety of ways that differ from what you are used to. Even if all you ever do is read your association's newsletter, it can be comforting to know that there are others out there who share your interests. Such a newsletter also gives you the opportunity to read articles on various aspects of the art.

If you make the effort to go to the events or workshops sponsored by an organization, it can also be a lot of fun to mix with the same students and instructors. Becoming a member can also lead to the opportunity to get involved in a range of administrative and organizational skills as needed to produce the events and workshops that are sponsored by such groups. Such skills can sometimes lead to better jobs in the "real world."

If the association has reasonably strict criteria for membership as well as grading, then you can also have the satisfaction and recognition that comes from having successfully completed the requirements for being a member in good standing or for having risen up the ranks of that organization.

The Bad Aspects

Martial and taiji associations are sometimes run by a particular clique or racial group and it can be difficult to find acceptance if you don't fit in in those ways. In addition, most such groups are nonprofit, volunteer-run associations, and these are notoriously inefficient at getting things done. Commonly, a few people end up carrying the ball and they tend to burn out as a result, which means a high turnover of volunteers and lack of organizational continuity.

In some organizations, egotistical, financial, stylistic, or racial infighting to control the activities of the group end up causing its premature dissolution. Or the founder resigns, retires, or dies and the organization he or she started falls apart for the same reasons when there is no longer either a firm hand in charge or a figurehead to inspire loyalty.

Sometimes the association itself is a thinly disguised money-making venture for a particular instructor or his system (e.g., buy a membership in a group headquartered in another city or country and you'll likely get nothing for your money except a membership certificate and the occasional bulletin). This is of particular concern to those living in the United States, as the American martial arts publications in particular are full of organizations with grandiose titles offering membership or meaningless certificates of rank for a small annual fee. These are the martial equivalent of the dubious institutions that sell college or university degrees to those who want to pad their business cards and resumes.

Ot course, it's your business if you want to pay a hefty price to someone you have never heard of in some obscure city to hang a certificate from the World Fighting Masters of Mystical Taijiquan on your wall, but it won't impress everyone as much as you may like!

Similarly, in regard to those associations that have little or no structure and no criteria for membership except buying a subscription to their newsletter or magazine, the more legitimate practitioner may find himself being judged unfairly by his peers for being part of such an association.

WHAT ABOUT SHORT SOLO FORMS?

I sometimes recommend the value of learning short or combined forms to experienced students as a way of broadening their understanding of whatever version of the traditional Yang style they may be studying. One such short form that I practiced with both enjoyment and benefit for several years was that developed and taught by William C.C. Chen of New York City.

That teacher's 60 Posture Form is a variation of the famous short form created by his even more famous teacher, Cheng Man Ching, who popularized taiji in the United States in the 1960s and early 1970s. William has been teaching continuously as long as I have been alive (since 1952), so it shouldn't be surprising that his insights and methods of practice should hold more than a little interest to those who are curious about how richly varied the Yang style can be.

The late Cheng Man Ching's famous 37 Posture Short Form is also worthy of study if you can find a good teacher in his lineage. On the other hand, many who don't care for his approach say that his short form is simply "watered-down taiji" aimed at lazy Westerners as he found them when he moved to New York in the 1960s. I don't think that an experienced practitioner will agree if he or she gets the chance to see the late master in some of the old films available of him demonstrating, or if he or she gets the chance to train under a few of his surviving students or their better disciples.

However, as is often the case with the real masters that you meet in modern times, part of Cheng Man Ching's overall skill came from personal genius and part of it came from years of hard training in a variety of martial systems and with a variety of traditional teachers. I guess what I am trying to say is that his short form was the expression of his experience and maturity in the same way that Sun Lu Tang's taiji form as well as Chen Pan Ling's combination form were the expression of their decades of research into xingyiquan, baguazhang, and taijiquan.

When a modern student learns such forms years after their creators have died, from students of students of those who first developed them, such study won't automatically bring anywhere near the same level of skill and understanding unless the intermediaries have something like their teacher's experience, physical martial skill, and wisdom. When this is not the case, they tend to end up with the shell of the form and not its substance.

I also believe that you should only learn any short form after you have considerable experience and some skill in one of the traditional versions of taijiquan. Unlike many modern teachers, I *do not* think that short forms are a good way to introduce beginners to a traditional taijiquan system. Too many of those same beginners will be too easily satisfied with, for example, the China Sport Committee 24 Posture Form developed as a way of "easing" modern students into a more serious practice.

Perhaps I'm not the best person to offer advice on this form, as it is about the only short form that I regret having learned, practiced, and taught in my early years of teaching. Aside from having been designed by a committee, it butchers the traditional sequence of moves, eliminates repetitions of some of the postures that are the most useful martially, and then puts in repetitions of snake creeps down, which is one of the least useful postures for combat. The latter posture also makes it much harder for beginners to train properly and safely.

The only instructors whom I have personally seen demonstrate this short form who make it look at all useful to a serious taijiquan practitioner are Liang Shou-yu and Sam Masich. But someone of their caliber can make pretty much any form—no matter how dismal—look better than it is. And no, I am not one of their students, although I have done workshops with both and greatly respect their skills and experience.

As I just suggested, part of the problem with short forms for those interested in learning about the martial skills that can be gained from studying the Yang style is that they are not only shortened versions of the originals, but have also often had the most useful martial postures removed or their useful martial sequencing scrambled. For example, techniques like wave hands in clouds, chop with fist, and step forward, parry, and punch, which get repeated often in the long set, are often done only once or not at all in the shorter versions or are not partnered with their correct prior or subsequent postures. In this regard, it is important to remember that the postures or techniques that are repeated the most in the long sequences are the ones that are the most useful and versatile in terms of martial efficacy!

I may be in the minority opinion, but I think that new recruits are always best served by learning the traditional forms and training methods in the proper order of doing so, as long as they have the health and interest to allow them to practice properly. A useful compromise for introducing the long, solo form to beginners is to teach the first section of that sequence as a self-contained form. In this way, as with the Reader's Digest condensed novels, the end product is still coherent although much shortened—the chapters and pages haven't been scrambled as well.

It remains good advice in taiji as in life to "start as you mean to go on!"

CAN YOU LEARN FROM INSTRUCTIONAL TAPES AND DVDS?

Like many aspects of the modern technological revolution, the proliferation of instructional videos on taijiquan, qigong, and related arts has been both beneficial and counterproductive. While the saying "the self-taught individual has a fool for an instructor" is certainly often true, it is equally true that studying any good instructor's products can be a legitimate, though challenging, way to improve your understanding of your chosen art.

Sadly, many who would like to try taijiquan classes don't have access to a good teacher and have little recourse except using video self-instruction, at least initially. There are always individuals who, through hard work or personal aptitude, can learn a great deal from such teaching aids. While it is difficult for most beginners to get more than a crude understanding of a particular form or training method from self-instruction, even a crude understanding is often better than nothing, as it can provide the springboard to motivate you to seek instruction from a real instructor.

While electronic instructional aides are more useful for the experienced student, even then such products are often most fruitful as a means of generating income for whoever produced them. Many of the instructors making videos are doing so specifically to augment their incomes and are less concerned about an accurate transmission of what they teach than they would be with their own personal students. For example, I have been told by more than one instructor over the years that they left errors on their video products to help sort out the students they meet who have only had this kind of instruction from those who have learned properly in other cities from legitimate representatives of that particular teacher.

In addition, the production costs of editing and reshooting scenes will often guarantee that minor mistakes are included in the final cut. Since real skill comes largely from being precise in your training, a few errors in that transmission may have surprisingly serious long-term results.

However, once you have achieved some skill under a teacher's watchful eye, it can also be very useful to study as many different videos as your time and budget will permit. This kind of study allows you to compare notes on the different ways of legitimately interpreting and teaching the forms and training methods.

As in all things, not all tapes and DVDs are created equal, and it is not always possible to identify a bad product until you have wasted your money. It is also important to remember that even a talented instructor can produce a video that is poorly lighted, hard to follow, and needlessly repetitious.

On the other hand, we tend to judge a product by its cost and this is not always appropriate. A lengthy, high-priced tape shot with fancy lighting and special effects may give you little of value, while a more modestly priced, hour-long product may deliver insights and instruction worthy of a lifetime of study. Similarly, don't automatically reject the tape produced by a martial unknown and assume that the one by the famous expert will necessarily be better.

If you are bewildered by the variety of videos available, try to rent copies of the ones that might interest you before buying. A few video rental outlets as well as bookstores rent such videos. You can also read the reviews that sometimes appear in the martial arts magazines and on martial arts discussion forums on the Internet. Such opinions are rarely impartial, but they are a starting point for comparison shopping.

When considering the purchase of a particular video, pay attention to whether it is a "demonstration" or "instructional" tape. A reputable producer or distributor will indicate which it is in the advertisements. The former are really only of use for comparison purposes or if you have learned the material in person and need a record for home study.

You should also realize that a tape or DVD produced in China, Hong Kong, or Taiwan may be labeled as instructional when it, by Western standards, it is hardly more detailed than a demonstration tape. Traditional teaching in the Orient was and is often done largely in relative silence. You copied the physical movements of the teacher to the best of your ability and that was that unless you were allowed to join the inner circle of senior students.

Tips on Learning with Videos

- Watch the entire tape or DVD through at least once before you start trying to learn any aspect of the training shown.
- If there is a recommended progression of how to learn on a particular tape, don't rush ahead or skip material that you think is familiar. If you have some relevant experience, it can be easy to convince yourself that you immediately understand the basics being taught on the screen. Such arrogance is usually self-defeating. Even though both activities involve knowing how to skate, is a hockey player also automatically qualified to be a figure skater and vice-versa?
- Be patient and take your time. If the on-screen instructor suggests that you learn no more than one move per week, then follow that advice. Proper study goes hand in hand with review—say every three months—especially of material that you already think you know. In the end, it's not making mistakes that is problematic.

We all make errors. The real error lies in failing to correct the mistakes you know about, from arrogance or plain laziness.

- If you are trying to learn push-hands or martial techniques, remember that you need a partner whom you practice with regularly to learn anything meaningful. Find a friend who wants to learn and train together. Two sets of eyes and brains are often better than one when it comes to figuring out how to interpret what seems so clear on the TV screen or computer monitor. (Of course, the downside of training with a friend is that you may start arguing with each other about who is interpreting the material correctly!)

It seems that many of those buying videos—no matter what their level of skill—watch them once or twice and then relegate them to a shelf without ever trying to practice, much less master, any of the forms or methods shown. However, many fine modern teachers have also been able to expand their audiences and spread the art by producing videos that can help long-distance students to get basic training to which they might otherwise never have been exposed.

This is particularly true if you make the opportunity to get periodic corrections or advice from someone who actually can do those same forms and methods with some competence. In the end, most of us will need this kind of correction, as it's much harder to fool yourself about your progress if, for example, someone tactfully reminds you that "your thumb doesn't go there" when you are demonstrating the toad in the hole qigong.

In fact, isn't seeing and evaluating yourself and your physical efforts accurately as you try to learn new skills one of the hardest skills to master, even when your teacher is there in the flesh?

Finally, please do not cut bootleg copies of an instructor's videos for yourself or your friends, or post such material on the Internet without getting written permission to do so. Infringing on copyright is stealing, no matter how creatively you rationalize it, and it cheapens the value of your efforts to learn.

SHOULD YOU CONTEMPLATE TEACHING?

There will come a time, if you train conscientiously enough, that you will probably have to come to terms with whether you want to teach classes of your own. There are several issues to consider:

- Teaching yet another group of beginners who don't look as if they can lift the TV remote control, much less remember tonight's lesson by the time that they get home, much less do any meaningful interactive training
- Trying to find the time and energy to practice for yourself after having spent too much time and energy teaching the basic forms and methods
- Maintaining your enthusiasm when only one or two students bother to make an appearance at a group class
- Being rained out or snowed under yet again on the time and day that your group meets outdoors even though it was sunny the rest of the week
- Having the community center where you teach combine what should be separate classes for beginners, intermediate, and advanced students into one class because of lack of enrollment in one or more of those levels without bothering to let you know ahead of time
- Having your classes taught at an office during lunch hour or after work unexpectedly moved into the foyer of the building "because we need the room for more important work"

- Having the martial arts school where you are teaching your taiji classes suddenly go bankrupt, thus depriving you of a place to teach even though your particular classes at that location had been going well

Whoops! Those are some of the many reasons I have experienced NOT to teach. Fortunately, there are also many good reasons to do so, though it should be obvious that I do have somewhat mixed feelings about the value of teaching Yang taijiquan after having done so since 1985 for anywhere from 9–25 hours per week and in a variety of spaces and formats continuously, except for a two-month period in which I was recovering from surgery.

Like many teachers I have met, I was originally thrust into that role by my own teacher at the time, who told me during a class to "go help the beginners." In traditional taiji classes, as it was with me, you may well be expected to teach those junior to you as part of the long-term learning process. Your interest in doing so is of less relevance than the wishes of the chief instructor. Sometimes, you may be able to say "No, thanks"—without repercussions—but in some clubs, doing this is a poor move in terms of continuing to get decent instruction afterward.

So let's assume that you have put in your time as a beginner and an intermediate level of student and that, after a few years, you have had some experience helping your instructor to coach the newer students and you find that you have some interest in or aptitude for teaching.

It's always courteous to ask your teacher if you have his or her permission to start classes on your own, as failing to do so with a more traditional teacher can have repercussions (being ignored from then on as part of his or her "taiji family" being the mildest and most common). In the old days, you wouldn't have dared to teach without the permission of a respected, long-term instructor. Today, for a variety of reasons, this is rarely the case.

Some teachers will insist on a well-defined financial relationship with you once you start to teach, especially if they are well known and you will be using their name in your advertisements. Some teachers will not care much one way or the other if you teach elsewhere as long as you continue to help out in their classes. Some teachers won't care much one way or the other, and some will encourage you to move somewhere else and start up your own classes to "spread the word!"

Deciding that you are ready and want to start teaching is one thing; adjusting to being the role model instead of a student is another. Learning to be a good teacher is like anything else in life: You have to have the basic skills, some aptitude, and put in the time to develop whatever teaching ability you can.

It is also a question of being patient, within reason, with your students' foibles and of teaching them each to the best of your ability on as much of an individual basis as the group size will allow. In the end, a few of those you teach over the years will blossom and most will either coast along or drop out. On the other hand, a good teacher can motivate at least some of the students to eventually do the same skills as well—if not better—as he or she.

Making money through teaching taijiquan isn't too hard; it's retaining your ethics as a practitioner and teacher that's the hard part. If you have a large school and overhead you'll need to advertise, which means you have to generate lots of beginners to pay for it, which means that you have to have either a number of qualified assistants to help you do the teaching, or large classes in which only the really talented will learn anything.

Now this is perhaps the rationalization of this poor businessman who has failed to achieve much financial success through his teaching. I will admit that I certainly always feel inadequate whenever I read the unsolicited infomercial magazines from American martial arts business organizations that promise that I can double my income by teaching summer camps to children and suggest that I am a failure if I am not following their financial advice.

Aside from wanting to teach to share what you know and perhaps earn an honest dollar or two while doing so, there is also the issue of sometimes having to create your own training partners to be able to practice the martial methods and forms. We live in a very mobile society and it is sometimes the case that you are thrust into having to teach privately or in small groups in a new city or town in order to have, eventually, someone worthwhile with whom to train in the interactive stuff.

In the end, running your own classes can "teach the teacher" many valuable lessons about your own understanding of the art. It is one thing to be able to do a form or training method or an entire system, but it is quite another to explain and demonstrate your performance in such a way that you help someone else to discover the same path that you have followed over the years.

PHYSICAL ISSUES

How Straight is Too Straight?

At the risk of making a bad pun, I would like to "articulate" my opinion on how straight the spine should be when doing the Yang style:

- Some experts say that the spine must be straightened to the point of "ironing out" the natural S-curve that nature intends us to have. They do this by tucking the tailbone in forcefully.
- Other experts say that the spine must be loosely straight with the minimal use of force and that twisting

the waist or hips is more important to power generation than the structure of the spine itself.

- Other experts say that the spine must be straight and firm but that the mingmen point on the spine in the lower back must act like a spring to provide a subtle but essential element to the generation of martial force.
- Other experts talk about lifting the head and having the spine and bones of the limbs and trunk "hang" from that structure as if they were relatively unimportant in comparison to the strength and rooting power of the legs.

My own take on the subject is that they are all correct to a certain extent and that the spine must be erect (as in relatively vertical) in order to make efficient and effective turning and twisting possible so as to direct the power of the legs and spine into the arms and hands. Conversely, if you manage to get access to old photos of the early Yang-style masters, it is obvious there was more leaning going on then than in later and modern versions.

I have been told more than once over the years that the slight lean inherent in the bow stance in the Yang style and the somewhat greater forward lean in the Wu-style bow stance is to generate "drop" to the impact that is generated by a practitioner. This is difficult to do properly in terms of the balance of the practitioner and this can be compromised by a target who moves out of the way at the last moment. It is also easier to over-bend the knees when leaning forward and this can have serious long-term ramifications for the health of those joints. My knees are fine after 30 odd years of taiji, but I can't say the same for many of the serious practitioners who I know.

Leaning properly without compromising balance is also done partly to make it easier for a taiji practitioner to slip the hands of an attacker over the top of the head if that person tried to grapple the neck or head. It is also true that "lift the back of the head, tuck the chin" is also crucial to slipping an attempt to get the hands around the base of the back of the skull. Many of the old postural requirements have as much to do with sound fighting fundamentals as anything else.

Perhaps the real problem is finding teachers who still understand these things or have rediscovered their martial usage.

However, if you keep the spine relatively straight, fold it primarily from the inguinal folds and not the waist, and have a connected springiness in the lower back and between the shoulder blades, then you'll be able to lean slightly forward or in any direction without compromising your balance and root.[1] Practice this against a variety of techniques and against a variety of partners and you will be able to understand how being straight is always essential and always relative and can't be learned through earnest discussions over the Internet or from a piece of paper.

Sadly, the average student will also find it is easier to become stiff while trying to be upright. Conversely, some will try to be so relaxed that they look as if they have been poured into a bowl. Their spines sag and hunch in a parody of good health while others will misread the classics and go to great effort to round the shoulders and tilt the pelvis.

The relatively vertical approach tends to hold up reasonably well in terms of modern sports science and any functional approach to efficient mechanics in the human body should have more similarities than differences. For example, competent basic standing yoga posture is almost identical to the posture recommended by someone who teaches the Alexander Method, as is that taught by a good taiji teacher. The latter is almost identical to the posture recommended by a good physiotherapist.

Keeping the spine vertical in its alignment between Heaven and Earth also has significance to certain traditionalists, as it makes it easier for the practitioner to act as a conduit for energy moving in a cyclic manner between those two sources of external qi. Even if you only approach it as a metaphor instead of literally, the old Chinese expression that "Heaven supports the Earth, Earth supports Man, and Man acts as the intermediary between Heaven and Earth" is a delightful way of describing the interrelationship of these aspects of life.

In fact, the relaxed straightness of the spine—whether it is held in a slight forward slant or vertically—is one of the most common linking factors in all the family styles of taijiquan as well as the other traditional internal martial systems.

As to tucking the tailbone under, there is a lot of nonsense in the modern internal arts that is a misinterpretation of old writings by translators who didn't have the technical skills necessary to do justice in English to the old sayings. One modern expert whom I respect greatly, who is both a skillful internal martial artist and a competent translator of Chinese, Tim Cartmell, suggests that the North American taiji obsession with tucking the tailbone and rounding and even hunching the chest at times results from a lack of good role models as well as not translating the relevant Chinese terminology properly.

Another modern expert whom I respect a great deal, Sam Masich, told me that he felt that the hunching and tucking of the upper torso that is often present in modern taiji is due to the influence of certain teachers of taiji who had also mastered southern kung fu styles that do this to generate power in certain ways. Teachers who had mastered those styles and later learned some taiji added aspects of their previous training to what they had learned about the Yang style in an attempt to reconcile the different approaches or just from having poorly understood the differences between the arts.

Particularly in North America and Europe, there seems to be a continuing trend in the Yang style to talk about keeping a straight spine and not leaning but actually to go out of the way to look round-shouldered and somewhat slumped in an attempt to be relaxed. Strange that it should be so, when you see photos of the old masters or recent well-trained immigrant teachers and the good ones are always very tall—no matter what their relative heights.

So perhaps it is excellent advice to remember your mother's constant urgings to "stand up straight!"

Is Yang-Style Taiji Good for Relieving Stress?

Most people who phone my studio to inquire about beginner-level taiji classes start the conversation by saying that they feel or have been told that they need to relax and they assume that taijiquan is the path to accomplish this. Very few such callers have even heard of the various family styles or know anything about taijiquan in real terms.

Occasionally, someone has done some reading or may have heard of the Chen style and knows that this is more demanding physically and more obviously martial, so they assume that Yang style is the "easy" one and that's what they want. Sadly, many also have been told that taiji is easy by well-meaning doctors and physiotherapists who also usually know little more about traditional taijiquan than their clients.

Many traditional Chinese doctors or massage therapists will also recommend that their clients learn taiji to improve their health and fitness levels. They are rarely talking about the older or martial versions of the Yang style, but rather those modern versions that are taught solely as a mild calisthenic or moving qigong. Of course, the postures and body mechanics required to do any style of taiji are relaxing in the sense that eventually relearning how to stand and move in accordance with the principles of the discipline will make you more efficient at both activities.

In physiological terms, real relaxation is related to creating postural integrity and encouraging deep abdominal breathing as well as loosening, strengthening, and stretching the body's connective tissue. In more traditional terms, accomplishing this kind of functional relaxation encourages the qi to be of a sufficient quality and quantity to flow in an unimpeded manner throughout the body.

However, in the beginning, relearning how to stand and move is anything but relaxing, either mentally or physically for most novices. This is because many beginners take up the Yang style because they are suffering from some chronic malady, have gotten out of the habit of regular exercise, or want to, above all, avoid stress. This is rather ironic as, in some ways, what most sedentary people could benefit the most from is more meaningful physical work in their daily lives—not more leisure time.

One of the living legends of the Yang style, Yang Zhen Duo, has done many workshops in North American in the last decade or so. He has gone out of his way through his translators to demonstrate and discuss how Westerners have wrongly assumed that taiji is about relaxation. His comments revolve around the concept that we have to think of relaxation as being one of many tools that are needed to understand the real reason for doing taiji: unifying the internal aspects of practice (use of the mind and breath), with the external (how to move and stand in accordance with the correct principles). Remember the six harmonies that were discussed in a previous chapter?

Even taking this good advice to heart, it is more likely that the first few months of classes will serve only to elevate the stress levels of the average beginner as he or she discovers that learning the Yang style is not as effortless as a good practitioner makes it look. Even with adequate and sincere instruction, a novice is more likely to leave even a solo form class tense and frustrated from all the demands put on him or her by the teacher or by his or her own need to feel that he or she is keeping up with the others in class.

Similarly, it is hardly easy for students to learn to apply the principles of posture and movement that they have learned through solo form to either a martial class or daily life. For example, even experts may have marvelous posture while training and then slump mindlessly while typing at a keyboard in front of a monitor.

Oh, and for those few interested in the martial side of taiji, don't assume that it is always a gentle exercise. Even when doing the milder versions of push-hands, it will probably be a shock for the average North American novice in terms of just how much effort is needed to do any of the martial exercises well. Many Western practitioners who have gone to the Orient on holiday or to study taiji are surprised to visit parks in the Orient and watch the locals, young and old, as they knock each other about in their push-hands play.

No matter how you approach your taiji training, shouldn't the highest expression of "being relaxed" be that you learn to maintain your physical balance and emotional calm while training in a stressful situation, and not just when doing form by yourself in a peaceful environment?

Is Yang Taiji Primarily a Healing or Martial Art?

There seem to be two major camps in North American Yang-style taijiquan. The adherents of the first believe that standing qigong or the long, slow form can heal just about any illness if the practitioner has enough faith. In this way the slow movements of the Yang style long form or standing qigong are primarily seen as being almost a supernatural means of meditating and self-healing.

By comparison, another group of teachers would argue that, with very few exceptions, there is no place for self-healing qigong methods in the traditional curriculum and that the long, slow form is not a type of self-healing qigong, as it is designed primarily to train martial energies. For these experts, your taiji training makes you fitter and stronger as a byproduct of the training—but is not the main goal of the training.

One of the delights of being an adult—also one of its hardships—is researching any subject well enough to make up your own mind on this and similar contentious issues.

Certainly the reputation of the founder of the Yang style, Yang Lu Chan, was not built on healing people but in defeating them. It sounds as if his personality was a harsh one as well, if even some of the stories that have come down to us are accurate. It's true that we shouldn't judge him from a modern perspective, as he was a product of a very different age and society. Perhaps, in light of the times that he lived in, he thought of himself and was considered by his peers to be a good person.

In any case, I have seen no evidence in almost 35 years of training and teaching the martial arts to contradict my impression that the health aspect of taiji (especially the Yang style) is anything but a relatively modern overlay on the art, even though it is now almost exclusively done for those reasons.

In this way, early teachers added traditional Chinese qigong or meditative techniques learned elsewhere to what they had learned of martial taiji in an effort to make the art more complete. Again, realistically, I don't think we'll ever know for sure. The older generation of teachers were too secretive, very little was put down in writing, and when it was it was often of most use to those already in the "know" (martial shorthand, so to speak).

In the long run, a good style of taijiquan, whether done as a martial art or for self-healing as a form of moving qigong, will make you a better and healthier person even if it cannot cure everything that may ail you. For example, in programatic terms, several research projects in the United States and in Canada over the last 20 years have shown what common sense should have suggested—that Yang-style slow form practice provides the same cardiovascular exercise value as walking at a moderate pace for an equivalent amount of time.

Modern research has also shown the benefit of any regular and moderate aerobic exercise, as in repetitively practicing the fast or weapons forms, for reducing the risk of stroke and heart attack as well as improving overall health levels and quality of life.

In the context of Western medicine, rhythmic exercise, by the alternate contraction and relaxation of muscles, improves circulation and avoids or minimizes the pain and fatigue caused by muscle tension. It accomplishes this primarily by dispersing accumulations of lactic acid (a byproduct of chemical energy production in the muscles) as well as by improving the efficiency of the lymphatic system.

As blood circulates throughout the body, fluid naturally leaks into tissue. A network of vessels known as the lymphatic system collects this fluid and returns it to the circulatory system. Like veins, lymph vessels contain valves to prevent a back-flow to form a one-way system. This system has no pump (in the way that the heart pumps the blood) and the collected fluids are moved exclusively through the action of muscular contractions. One of the main benefits of twisting the waist and exercising the body to maintain muscle strength and tone as is found in taiji is the beneficial effect that this has on the normal functioning of the lymphatic system.

In addition, this system is important to the immune system, as it filters and produces infection-fighting white blood cells called lymphocytes. When the main ducts of the system are blocked or damaged, a large amount of lymph can quickly accumulate and cause serious edema, which in turn can cause several serious medical conditions.

It is also true, particularly for older students, that doing the long, slow form also provides a relatively gentle weight-bearing exercise that can slow or prevent osteoporosis, particularly in women.

In fact, it is one of the paradoxes of modern training that students can and do sometimes achieve dramatic self-healing from simply believing that the practice of taiji can heal them. I have seen it in my own students over the decades. Even stranger (and perhaps most frustrating for those trying to teach quality taijiquan), I have also seen people who have clearly improved their health and achieved some measure of inner peace by practicing debased forms taught by charismatic teachers who anyone else would have called charlatans.

I suppose that we shouldn't be surprised that this can happen, as it is simply another example of Cheng Man Ching's comment on how his students "didn't have enough faith." Indeed, the mind and faith, even when misplaced, can achieve miracles. In recent years, Western doctors have become more willing to admit that the placebo effect (i.e., believing that a treatment will heal you) is a powerful ingredient in many cures. It has been shown that the subconscious mind and emotional stress can make a person sick. Why is it such a hard leap of faith to see the reverse, that the mind and faith in a method can actually heal?

Training in taijiquan is hardly a quick fix for any chronic, much less acute, disease or injury. It is also essential to understand that lifestyle changes are an inevitable and essential aspect of improving one's health.

As the training starts to sink in, and perhaps much to your own surprise, you may find yourself wanting to quit smoking in a way that you may never have experienced before, or you may find that you don't get the same number of episodes of the flu or colds in winter, or it may seem gross to eat fried or fatty foods, or you may find yourself less stressed by certain things than used to drive you up the wall.

However, change is a funny thing, whether you are trying to do it or it just seems to happen over time. We may consciously think we want to improve ourselves or get rid of bad habits and then subconsciously resist doing so, or grieve for the fact that we have lost interest in our old ways of behaving.

I think it is also fair to say that seriously studying taijiquan can increase the pace at which one matures. As the years roll by and your skill levels in and understanding of the Yang style improve, your priorities and interests will change. What was important at age 25 (e.g., developing physical skill, learning self-defense skills, or becoming a better fighter) will be less important at age 40 or 50.

Assuming that you have shown some aptitude and have practicing regularly, this is partly a reflection of the fact that you will have improved your health and also achieved real self-defense skills. By middle age, your skills should have reached the point that the arts no longer are a major focus—an obsession—but simply an important aspect of your daily life. You have come to terms with both your skills and limitations as a practitioner and learned to value your daily training for its own sake, not just as a vehicle for self-improvement or good health.

However, time and experience also play an essential part in whether or not you are still reacting like a child to all of life's tribulations by the time you are middle-aged. There is real magic in competent instruction and diligent practice over the long term, but it is hardly a miracle cure for all of our physical and emotional problems. Coming to terms with this is also part and parcel of the maturing process as a practitioner.

We all want miracles. Even those who seem the most cynical want to feel as if they are tapping into something special. It's very hard to come to terms with the issue of both skill and wisdom coming only through long-term effort. In particular, the martial skills can only be purchased through a credit card issued by the Bank of Blood, Sweat, and Tears.

In the end, being fit and strong in martial terms as well as being relatively relaxed and calm can certainly improve your physical and emotional life, but common sense should tell you that you remain mortal no matter how skillful you are at any aspect of taijiquan—which leads us to the next controversial topic.

Does Taiji Make Me Immune to Normal Wear and Tear?

Perhaps because of the New Age veneer on many of the North American variations of taiji (particularly, but not exclusively, the Yang style), there tends to be an expectation in both students and teachers that somehow regular practice will eliminate most if not all physical ills and somehow confer immunity to illness and general physical wear and tear.

More than once, prior to my having hip-replacment surgery in 2005, I had people say to me "How come you had osteoarthritis in your hip when you practice taiji?" I have also been told many times by students during the flu and cold season, "I thought I wouldn't get sick if I practiced taiji regularly."

Of course, this kind of unrealistic attitude is not unique to the Yang style. Some years ago, a friend of mine who taught Reiki developed cancer. Coming to terms with the disease and the loss of a breast was hard enough, but she also had to deal with several supposed friends who accused her of being a fraud in the arts that she loved so much because she had become ill with cancer. The implication was clear: She must "deserve" to be sick and she must not have mastered her own healing arts!

In addition to such stupid prejudice, taiji forms and methods that are taught without proper attention to body mechanics and the student's health limitations can also cause a variety of physical trauma. The most common physical complaints that I hear from my colleagues, as well as long term practitioners, is chronic pain in the knees or shoulders.

The causes vary according to the variety of taiji and the various strengths and weaknesses of the individual practitioners, but the overall truth is simply that taiji is much more demanding than it looks. Those who practice are liable to wear out parts of their bodies in doing so over the decades. It is also hard to come to terms with the fact that it simply takes longer to recover from even minor injuries as one goes through middle age.

The knee is often the first joint to go and improper kicking methods are often to blame, especially if you are kicking too slowly or too high and straining the joint that way, or if you are doing fast kicks into the air so that the joint is repeatedly hyperextending to a greater or lesser degree. Pain and damage can also be caused by practicing forms that use extended bow stances and require or ignore that you are overbending the knee of the weighted leg.

Similarly, if your style uses weighted turns, those are easily done incorrectly and torque the knee joint repetitively. Sometimes, you may well be doing it perfectly on the right side and not even realizing that the left isn't doing the same thing.

If you are overweight or sedentary before starting your taiji training, you are even more likely to stress your knees or lower back if your posture and body mechanics are not adequate to the demands of your standing or moving activities. It is a good thing to practice forms or training methods in such a way that you don't favor (and overwork) your dominant side.

One way around this is to learn or teach yourself the mirror-image version of whatever you practice regularly so that you work your body evenly. Unfortunately, it also makes more sense to practice the martial techniques that you like the best to favor your dominant side, rather than wasting time trying to do each technique equally well from both a "righty" and a "lefty" perspective.

The traditional forms don't tend to be evenly balanced except in those postures that are particularly useful from a fighting perspective. This should tell us what these internal forms were originally designed to do! They weren't mechanisms for getting in touch with your inner child.

For those of us who train seriously, year after year, in the martial side of the art, there's also the price of contact injuries, both chronic and acute. For example, I have arthritis in both elbows from being a training partner for too many students who didn't have the control that prevents needless damage.

I learned the hard way why many instructors rarely trained with the beginner and intermediate students—too much risk of injury from students with too much enthusiasm and not enough control. Sadly, those are exactly the students who need to feel the teacher's skill and power the most.

By the way, those students who don't practice as regularly on their own often have much less chance of developing serious training-related injuries of either the acute or chronic varieties than those who train with dedication and regularity. One of life's little ironies is that one of the rewards for diligence is a greater chance of suffering physically for your efforts.

Everyone should practice moderately and not neglect getting warmed up and stretched (the two activities are not the same) before *and* after training, as well as paying attention to doing the forms and training methods to the best of your ability at that point in your development. Many injuries come from being inattentive of proper body mechanics or of overdoing the training itself.

The length of each of your training sessions and their frequency in your schedule depend on a number of variables: your own level of interest, physical ability, time constraints, etc. For example, one or two hours of classroom instruction per week can be sufficient over the long term for learning the long, slow form, if it is bolstered by daily solo practice. On the other hand, martial competence will require much more frequent attendance at a private or group class before the basic skills start to sink in, as they can only be learned through interactive as opposed to solo practice.

It is also probably true that few modern teachers, much less their students, practice with the intensity that the old masters brought to their training. Of course, the latter had to be skilled at a variety of forms, training methods, and even archaic weapons, as they never knew when they would be challenged by a rival. Few adults with families or occupations can match such training regimens, but it remains true that regular practice is essential to making progress—especially if your interest goes beyond doing this discipline as more than a set of physical movements.

Once a day should be the bare minimum if you hope to see any real benefits on a self-healing basis from the practice of the long, slow form. As I like to repeat to my students, practicing standing qigong, preferably for a minimum of 15 to 30 minutes on a daily basis, is also an essential aspect of serious study, at least for the first few years. If you are training in solo versions of the fast or weapons forms, these must also be fitted into your schedule on a regular basis.

As I have previously suggested, practicing on a variety of types of targets is essential to learning about striking with the hands, elbows, knees, and feet. However, in recent years I have come to think that it is better to tone down the expression of power (i.e., fajing) while training forms and save it for when you are hitting a striking surfaces that help absorb some of the power being generated. Shadow boxing is essential, but not at full power—especially when you are no longer young.

By the way, modern research has shown that the traditionalists were on the right track about the morning and evening being the best times to practice. People are more inclined to skip scheduled exercise in the middle to late afternoon because of fatigue or busy schedules. For slower or steadier exercise, like slow form, jogging, or bicycling, you'll reap the same benefits whether you practice early or late in the day. However, high-intensity activity, like repetitive practice of fast forms that requires short bursts of energy, are best done late in the day. You'll feel stronger, perform more skillfully, and get more out of your workout, according to Dr. David W. Hill, a professor of kinesiology, in a study released in 1993 at the University of North Texas.

The self-healing and defense skills of taijiquan are gained gradually through moderate and balanced training. The obsessive younger student may quickly develop martial skills to some extent, but lose out in other ways by upsetting the balance in his or her daily life. Conversely, the older obsessive student may train too hard initially and get injured by trying too hard or beyond his or her age-related limitations. Similarly, the lackadaisical student trains only when the mood takes him or her and then overinflates the value of such training, or gets discouraged because practicing and attending class once a week doesn't seem to be producing noticeable benefits.

Finally, the last bit of advice that I can offer is to the one that I have the hardest time following personally. If you have injured yourself or start suffering from chronic pain in some part of the body, have it evaluated and treated by a qualified Western doctor, a physiotherapist, or a qualified Traditional Chinese Medicine (TCM) doctor.

Don't pretend that everything is fine when you are obviously suffering from new acute or chronic conditions, or pain that is likely related to your training. And do not ask your teacher for medical advice unless he or she happens to be one of the above!

Fit or Fat?

A disturbing trend in modern Yang-style taiji is the number of people who practice with some competence but think that being potbellied or seriously overweight is somehow a sign that they have achieved true "softness." Similarly, many modern Yang-style teachers have a strange attitude to cardiovascular exercise and don't tend to value it as much as a modern personal trainer or athlete will.

It is true that being very fit from a cardiovascular perspective doesn't guarantee that you won't die an early death from heart troubles. Of course, not having any cardiovascular endurance can also shorten your life, so perhaps the real answer still remains elusive.

On the subject of hearts, I remember a few years ago an American medical study that speculated that the human organism is born with a certain number of total heartbeats programmed into it, and that when your allotment of beats expired, you did as well. If true, that would indicate the Daoists were ahead of their time indeed to suggest that any hard exercise that makes your heart beat much faster than normal for sustained periods would only shorten your ordained lifespan.

However, modern students are more often suffering from having no exercise program. It should be obvious that being or becoming healthy and fit through your training is desirable and will allow you to make progress faster than an unfit student who remains that way. However, common sense sometimes goes out the window in the modern internal martial arts. There seems to be a common misconception in North American taijiquan in particular that it is not necessary to be physically fit to do the Yang style, as the system focuses on being "soft."

In this way, students are told or assume that activities like yoga, weight lifting, and cardiovascular training are not only superfluous to your daily routine, but actually counterproductive to making progress. As a result of this not uncommon attitude, there seem to be a disproportionate number of potbellied, overweight teachers and students at North American workshops and taiji events.

I once read an article by an outspoken taiji instructor (a "lean and dour" Scot named Dan Docherty) who wrote that his first and most lasting impression of an American taiji event that he attended was that it was the largest collection of overweight, middle-aged, and balding men with ponytails that he had ever witnessed.

Being heavy doesn't imply that you have learned some secret of the Yang style because you have achieved the same build as the legendary Yang Cheng-fu, who was more than 6 feet tall and almost 300 pounds in his later years. It's important to remember that he died rather young and that his obesity was perhaps a factor in that early death.

I think part of the problem lies in the fact that competition style push-hands often is won by those practitioners who are heavy because it is easier for them to manipulate a lighter opponent, especially if really low stances are used. In martial terms, size does matter and it isn't a surprise that Sumo wrestlers are huge in size. Again, it also isn't a surprise that most of them retire early due to obesity-related health issues.

Perhaps because it attracts older, middle-class students in North America, there is a tendency in such classes to work only as the mood takes you and to spend more time sipping tea and discussing theory or gossiping about your classmates.

Similarly, I also find it difficult to be patient with those practitioners whom I meet who obviously believe that doing a short form variation of the Yang style for a few minutes a few times a week somehow automatically makes them superior, in every way, to someone who does cardiovascular sports or trains regularly and intensively in one of the external martial arts.

May I suggest that if your teacher has lousy posture, is 40 pounds overweight, huffs and puffs after a few seconds of demonstrating fast form, and sneers at those who lift weights or do cardiovascular exercise, that you should go to the nearest exit if you are serious about your Yang style training?

Granted, you don't have to be either young or an athlete to be an effective fighter in self-defense terms, but it is equally silly to assume that your training should not increase your strength and overall health while improving your posture. Staying in a counterproductive taiji environment is like going to a seriously obese doctor who wheezes at you, "You need to stop smoking, lose weight, and get some exercise," as he reaches for another Twinkie with nicotine-stained hands.

Do the Hands Lead or Does the Waist Lead?

The general rule of thumb in the Yang style is that the power is rooted in the feet, channeled through the legs, directed by the waist and mind, and expressed in the hands, which would imply that the hands are the final link in the chain.

Unfortunately, it is not as clear-cut as that in the sense that it is essential in martial terms that the body does not get there too much ahead of the hands. A good fighter will hit you immediately if you are within his range and your face or torso rush ahead of your hands and feet. "Leading with your face" is never a good idea martially.

Aside from such immediate practical considerations, the hands must lead in practical terms, as they must make contact initially both to "sense" where the opponent's body is as well as stick to and neutralize whatever he is trying to do to you while you launch your own attacks.

This does not refer to the common martial situation in which you crudely lead with your fist to strike someone, as is likely to happen when you confuse the need to get your fist into the target with the need to get your body weight to power the strike rather than lag behind.

Some good variations of the Yang style that I have experienced and seen not only teach that the hands must lead the weight of the body, but some good teachers also say that the hands must pull the body into position. This seems to contradict that the waist and weight changes must always lead the hands.

I have also read and been told more than once over the years that in the older versions of the Chen style, the first form uses the waist to lead the hands and the second (which is faster and more vigorous) has the hands leading the body.

I have found in my own practice and teaching that my hands will often feel as if they are pulling the rest of me toward whatever targets are accessible at that moment. This is usually triggered when using a more up-and-down, whole-body power.

There are references to the desirability of the hands leading the body in other internal systems in which this action is likened to the way that a monkey climbs a vine hand over hand and pulls itself upward and forward that way. I sometimes call this "pulling yourself up the bannister" power to make it clearer to my students. It can work particularly well in close-range grappling and controlling situations.

In the end, it is always the coordination of a well-trained body that will allow the hands and feet to support each other successfully in martial terms.

How Slow is Too Slow? How Fast is Too Fast?

The Yang style in particular, and taiji in general, is famous partly because the forms are normally done more slowly than the other Chinese martial arts, or relatively slowly with a few fast moves interspersed. One of the reasons that modern Yang style is so popular is that moving slowly and carefully is very relevant to elderly or infirm beginners or those who are unused to regular physical activity.

However, the origins of taiji art are unquestioningly martial, so there must have been an original reason for the relative slowness of the forms compared to the fast and furious pace that are normally part and parcel of hard style training. The answer is simple enough—moving relatively slowly allows you to be precise in your movements and to pay attention to the details of posture and body mechanics that tend to disappear when the forms are done quickly right from the start. Momentum and velocity can cover up a multitude of technical sins, especially in terms of balance and coordination.

It is also true that some Yang teachers advocate practicing the slow form as slowly as possible to try and turn the solo practice into a form of moving qigong that also trains a very deep root and challenges the legs in terms of muscular development.

While it can certainly be difficult to train yourself to do the long form at a 45-minute pace, I'm not sure that you will really benefit more than someone who does it a 30-minute pace. It is also true that the slower you go, the more likely you are to stop here and there in the form (which most Yang style teachers consider a "no-no") as well as putting a needless strain on your legs, particularly the knees and hips, in doing so.

In the spirit of moderation, I tell my students to practice the long, slow form at an even pace that seems natural to them with a minimum of 20 minutes for one round of practice and a maximum of 30–45 minutes for doing it slowly, depending on their age, physical strength, and experience.

In this regard, it is important to remember that the goal of partner training—for a long time—is to match his or her speed. This is an important concept, as being faster than your partner or opponent is not necessarily superior if your hands move so fast that your timing is affected and you are moving too fast to defend properly. This is less obviously a problem than moving too slowly, as even the most lackluster martial beginner will immediately realize that his hands are too slow if the attack he reacted to outpaces his defense.

Practicing at the same pace as your partner begins to build timing skills because matching someone else's pace is quite tricky—especially if that pace varies subtly or grossly. In the long run, more advanced applications of this slow/fast expression of yin/yang mean that you can break an opponent's timing to dominate with your own. But such ideas are outside basic training.

The two-person application and weapons sets should be performed more quickly and at a variety of paces, as it is important to remember that while moving slowly is essential training in taiji, it is also not a substitute for fast training when such is appropriate. Maintaining correct posture and body mechanics is not much easier to do quickly and the forms can become a way of training quickness and also provide cardiovascular conditioning. Remember the idea of yin *and* yang, slow *and* fast, soft *and* hard?

Sexuality and Taiji Training

Gender-related issues can also cause problems in a modern mixed training environment. This wasn't a problem in the good old days in China, as there weren't any mixed classes. Women learned only from their fathers, brothers, or husbands, if they were lucky enough to have one who was also an instructor. In more recent years, in government-run martial arts colleges on the Mainland, women experts teach form and qigong to women, but rarely the combative aspects of the art and rarely in a mixed class.

While this is sexist in modern Western terms, it also avoided issues that often come up in modern classes: those looking more for new romantic or sexual partners than for quality taiji and, in the martial classes, those men who feel that they can fondle female students under the pretense of having accidentally made contact during the various two-person exercises.

In regards to the latter, both sexes must be prepared for the intimacy of many of the two-person training methods and for accidental contact with certain tender parts of each other's anatomy. To make this whole issue more complicated, In traditional terms, arousal (as in the emotional and physical intimacy that can develop when training with a partner of the opposite sex) does increase the production of sexual hormones, which can be refined through your training into martial or self-healing qi. It is also just as liable to lead to something a little more intimately mundane.

Human beings are sensual and tactile by nature. Enjoying the feel of another person's body as you practice is part of the pleasure of training—like dancing with a good partner. It doesn't mean that you're debauched to feel this way; however, you mustn't carry it too far the other way, either. Push-hands or grappling shouldn't be allowed to become foreplay.

One well-known American taiji intructor summed it up nicely at a post-workshop dinner that I attended in his honor many years ago. When asked by an attendee what he thought of Daoist sexual theory and practices, as well as I can remember it, he replied, "People like to have sex and Daoist practices are as good an excuse as any."

In addition, in terms of developing self-defense skills, women are usually going to be at risk from a larger man as, sexual-dominance issues aside, aggressors are often compensating for their own cowardice by looking for smaller victims. Consequently, women should practice with men, at least some of the time, to develop skills that might actually work on the street against male aggressors.

Despite what some instructors may piously suggest, size does matter when it comes to learning how to defend yourself. The techniques that work against someone your height and weight may fail miserably against someone much taller and heavier. By the way, in terms of developing pure self-defense skills, my publisher, Paladin Press, has put out a large variety of instructional books and videos that address the problem of practical self-defense. Some are written by and aimed specifically at women.

In addition, as a close-range system, many of the techniques of the Yang style require that the whole body be used as part of the delivery mechanism so that there is no choice about having an arm pinned across the chest on occasion.

Not every woman will want to do this type of technique and, even if she does not mind, may find it painful. Conversely, not every male student will feel comfortable about having his arm pinned across a woman.

It can also be difficult for women to get the idea of defending the chest, as men will often avoid contact with the breasts (and they should), but that means that the woman will never learn to deal properly with incursions into that area. This is also an issue when two women train together, as they will still avoid the area of the breasts. While it is not the only solution, it is an option for a woman studying push-hands or the more vigorous martial skills to get into the habit of wearing either a chest protector or one of the sparring bras that have plastic cups. Although, to be frank, I find that very few women find them comfortable or want to wear them in the same way that most male students ignore the common sense of wearing an athletic support and protective cup.

As in most aspects of trying to adapt traditional methods to modern needs, it is not easy to avoid diluting the martial content of taijiquan as the easiest way of avoiding controversy. It is certainly in the best interests of each instructor, from both a liability and ethical point of view, to outline to his or her students what is and isn't appropriate in terms of practicing push-hands in a mixed environment. However, it's difficult to supervise a group class from the point of view of what is too much or "sexist" contact. One person may be completely unaware of contact that might make another extremely uncomfortable.

In this regard, I remember a taiji workshop that I attended years ago in which one of the students who had accompanied me, a rather reserved and quiet man, was doing touchy-feely push-hands with an attractive middle-aged "hippie" type woman. He was so obviously doing his best to avoid her breasts in the exchange that I guess she got tired of being treated this way. She took one of his hands and put it on her right breast and said to him, "Don't worry about it." I happened to be watching when this happened and the look on my student's face was priceless!

However, not everyone is as comfortable as she was with intimate contact. I don't think that it is a valid solution to split group classes into male-only and female-only, however, as this may eliminate some problems but create new ones. For example, some people aren't comfortable with being touched by people of the same sex or, conversely, like it very much.

As in most aspects of trying to adapt traditional methods to modern needs, it is not easy to avoid diluting the martial content of taijiquan as the easiest way of avoiding controversy. Instructors must be willing to be flexible and, in the end, this may mean limiting the techniques practiced in a group setting where supervision is "spotty" due to numbers or ensuring that women work only with women and men only with men. Aside from training issues, the sexual issues go deeper, as I have also met more than one taiji teacher who claims to teach the secrets of "dual cultivation" of sexual energies (a legitimate though rare and controversial aspect of qigong/religious Daoism). Charismatic and unscrupulous teachers use their reinterpretation of these sexual practices as a way to entice new sexual partners from among their students.

These are not always willing, and it is a sad aspect of modern martial arts training that, in recent years, more than one high-profile instructor has been charged by the police for interfering sexually with his much younger students during such private sessions.

Even more have not crossed the lines on a legal level, but have used their positions to seduce one sexual partner after another. Even when the students seem willing enough, it is an abuse of authority to seduce a student who may have an unhealthy adulation for his or her teacher. There are always those who are attracted to authority figures for a variety of reasons. Unscrupulous teachers frequently have no trouble leading them astray.

It is also true that some teachers will be at risk of having their innocent intentions misread and of being accused of things that have never even entered their minds. It is perhaps an indication of the complexity of our politically correct times that a male instructor who I knew would not do private classes with female students because he had been falsely accused of sexual harassment, but then got harassed and accused of sexist attitudes because he refused to teach women!

Some practitioners also are told or believe that sexual abstinence is essential for being healthy and cultivating qi. This is one aspect of traditional Chinese training. Abstinence as a way of purifying the Daoist or Buddhist monk and or the warrior is an age-old tradition in both Eastern and Western culture (the Knights Templar and the Knights of St. John are examples of medieval European attempts to unite the two concepts).

This agenda also often gets carried to ridiculous extremes by those with a sexual or emotional ax to grind. There is also the issue of refraining from sexual pleasure as a way of retaining your vital fluids to preserve your health. This concept crosses many cultures and is a common enough belief even among modern athletes.

Actually, I suspect that the venerable Oriental approaches to preventing or controlling male ejaculation may have had more to do with older rich men trying to keep up with the needs of a household with several wives and concubines! It's also always a good idea to introduce common sense when faced with extreme views on human sexuality. Remember that even Sigmund Freud was quoted as saying, "Sometimes a cigar is just a cigar."

Many famous and not-so famous taiji teachers who I have met have been fond of female company and have continued to demonstrate that interest into old age. Their spirit and qi are still vital although the body grows old.

It is also relevant to point out that many of the best Chinese masters that I have met were also heavy drinkers, heavy smokers, ate whatever food was put in front of them, and argued with their wives, girlfriends, and children—in other words, they were ordinary human beings, warts and all. You rarely do your teacher a favor by putting him or her up on a pedestal—there are too many temptations that can lead to a fall.

MARTIAL ISSUES

What Makes a System "Internal"?

Those few modern experts that you meet in the Yang style who actually have some legitimate claim to practicing their martial art in an internal manner will tell you that their doing so is the product of long years of difficult training. The better ones rarely make fun of their external arts peers or think that what they are practicing or teaching is innately superior to that being done by other good practitioners.

As I mentioned in an earlier chapter, styles commonly referred to as internal (taijiquan, baguazhang, xingyiquan, and the Wudang systems, among others) are based primarily on the understanding of not applying force directly against force, as well as using the power of the body as a coordinated whole to exploit the weaknesses of an opponent's technique or posture. By contrast, the external styles will often rely on overconditioning parts of the body and will base their defenses on their technical abilities to attack, regardless of the punishment that they absorb while doing so.

A popular source of discussion on the various taiji and martial arts boards is whether such a distinction is too artificial. I think that there is some truth to this contention, as it is important to remember that, prior to the 20th century, all-Chinese systems were generally referred to simply as martial or fighting arts. The stylistic distinction between internal and external was popularized by a few martial artists and writers in the late 19th and early 20th centuries for a variety of ideological and social reasons, e.g., wanting to differentiate between arts that were native to China (Daoist) from those that were foreign (Buddhist, Tibetan, Manchurian, European) in origin.[2]

Of course, for many practitioners, being "internal" is an intellectual label that they wrap around their pretentiousness, and not a particular set of physical abilities that can be applied both in solo practice and with others. In addition, each stylistic variation of the internal arts will identify those physical abilities in slightly or greatly different ways

I stopped doing demonstrations years ago and don't talk about "internal" versus "external" as much as I used to for a variety of reasons. Part of that reluctance is that I got tired of feeling like a trained monkey who was willing to perform for anyone with a few peanuts or coins. Part of that reluctance is also that martial ability is martial ability, and most modern internal arts practitioners have little, if any, combative abilities.

In the end, it is important that doing your martial training in an internal manner be both an expression of mastery through effort, dedication, and perseverance, and a factor of finding a legitimate expression of whatever systems you study and then doing your best to follow their principles to the best of you ability. Otherwise, your fighting or body movement may be effective for combat or be pleasurable for you to practice, but it won't necessarily be an expression of the Yang style.

In the end, the true meaning of being "internal" is up to each practitioner to define in terms of their own needs. I recommend the words of Ezra Pound, who wrote, in *ABC of Reading,* "Real education must ultimately be limited to men who insist on knowing: the rest is mere sheepherding."

Is Yang-Style Taijiquan Good for Self-Defense?

There are times when I get frustrated by the present state of the Yang style and have to agree with Erle Montaigue, who was often heard to answer "no" when people asked him if the Yang style was a good martial system. This despite the fact that he is one of the most competent martial artists that I have met in the Yang-style world. I think the comment is more a reflection of his frustration over how low this great system has fallen in recent years as a way of training combative skills.

I understand his sentiments, as after you have watched a few demonstrations of overweight, aging instructors resisting being pushed on stage by an equally overweight line of students, or seen an elderly teacher wave his hands from a distance only to have his "attackers" start bouncing up and down or falling over while still many feet away, it is hard to stay calm about the issue.

Most serious taiji students have read or been told stories about the old master who passively allows himself to be beaten by a gang of ruffians. When they leave, he gets up as if nothing had happened while, over the following days, the ruffians are all incapacitated by injuries caused by the beating they thought they were inflicting on their victim. Having had the experience of striking a modern-day expert or two with stiff force when I was a relative beginner, only to have it rebound painfully into my limbs, I will admit that there may well be something in such old tales.

However, most of us aren't capable of such marvelous demonstrations of passive resistance. The same can be said of occasional depiction of taiji in the Chinese cinema in which the stereotypical elderly master stands immobile and resists effortlessly the pushing of many younger attackers, or who pushes somebody effortlessly "many tens of feet away."

In a real fight, at the risk of shattering such illusions, success is more likely to favor those who blend offensive and defensive tactics and don't just hope to rely on being totally on the defensive through the skills of neutralizing and yielding. Such tactics are unlikely to work against skillful aggression if that's all you have trained to do with cooperative partners.

Sadly, a street fight is not always won by the good guy or the one who relies only on the skills used in the relative safety of modern push-hands competitions. In a real fight, the first one or two effective techniques usually decide who is the victim and who is the victor and, unlike the movies and competitions between trained martial athletes, where fights go on, and on, and on, real violence tends to start and be over almost before you can analyze what is happening.

Kicks are rarely used unless with an element of surprise or to finish someone who has been knocked down. If you're not ready for such events (both psychologically as well as in terms of being hit), the first contact may injure or shock you enough to leave you open to subsequent blows.

However, you also can't count on your first strike—no matter how precise and powerful—stopping a determined aggressor, as there are many people who act as if hitting them with considerable power just serves to throw the switch that activates their fighting ability. Over the years, I have seen a small man hit in the head with a real wooden chair who didn't even blink as he kept charging. I have seen someone else hit in the groin with a full-power kick who still had the rage to flatten the fellow who kicked him before himself collapsing in pain. No matter how skillful you are, you can never tell how your target will react until it is almost too late.

Alcohol and drug use may well slow down a fighter's reactions to your advantage but, this also makes him or her impervious to superficial pain and may temporarily give that person maniacal strength.

Similarly, no one, no matter what their skill level, knows how he or she will react until faced with real danger the first time, as opposed to sparring with an opponent in a friendly competition or with a fellow student in the safety of your training environment.

In other words, you can't plan how you will fight, because a fight is a fast, sloppy, and totally unpredictable event with variables as wild as weather conditions affecting the pavement you must stand on to defend yourself, or wearing clothing in winter that affect how easily and effectively you can move your limbs.

If you want to maximize your self-defense potential, you have to practice accordingly. In combat terms, relaxation means not panicking if struck or suddenly forced to fight and being able to work in close contact with the attacker without being immediately grappled or thrown, which implies staying physically balanced and using effective tactics *immediately.*

My main teachers both told me the same thing over the years : The methods should give you basic self-defense skills in a few months or years, but refining those skills will take a lifetime of ongoing effort. Over the decades, I have found this to be true—and so have many of my students. Short-term skills are rough and involve the risk of bruises (to the ego and elsewhere) and a substantial amount of sweat. The beginning of the forging process, so to speak.

Since beginning to teach taiji, I am happy to say that I have not had to fight anyone. However, I had some relevant experiences in my younger days and in more recent years have maneuvered my way out of a few situations that could easily have become ugly if I had panicked or overreacted. In addition, I have witnessed a number of street fights; this kind of real violence tends to spring out of nowhere. Sadly, you can't always avoid trouble by avoiding bars, drunken young people, and bad areas. Many muggings and acts of random violence occur when and where you least expect them. However, in general, it is relatively easy to avoid most situations that could lead to a fight unless you live in a high-crime area. (It is also true that police statistics reveal that most reported assaults and fights are with someone who the victim knows or lives with. Perhaps a course in anger management or mediation would be more useful than the average taiji class for developing self-defense skills for the average adult.)

Being shoved or hit in anger by someone who is stiff, untrained, and relatively uncommitted to hurting you can be much easier to deal with if you can relax even marginally more than your opponent and have some martial skill. However, stiffness combined with superior size, rage, or skill is a different proposition and one not usually met when training in a classroom setting. It is best to train with the worst opponent in mind and not the easiest.

Those who like to fight "for fun" and do so routinely are very dangerous opponents—much more so than most recreational martial artists that I have met. In fact, those who enjoy fighting and do so regularly don't tend to be ridiculously stiff opponents, as they enjoy or have grown used to close contact. It is unlikely that anyone would be able to depend on their superior relaxation or jing skills—if that's all they have—to do anything useful against such a person, with the kind of skills developed solely through push-hands.

Those practitioners who never experience anything other than cooperative training tend to get a very false sense of what happens in even the crudest and stupidest of self-defense scenarios. The short answer is that unrehearsed contact training (light to full contact) is essential to martial training with any pretense of reality. While such training doesn't have to have the intensity that competitive sports fighters prefer and are capable of, it does have to be present in some way, in some of your martial training time, if you want to claim that your skills have the potential for self-defense.

In my limited experience, even a seasoned recreational martial artist can fall apart as soon as you move into him or her at close range and without telegraphing your intentions. Some of the experiences that I have had when teaching new students who were experienced recreational martial artists over the years would be hilarious if they didn't also highlight how hard it is to translate modern taiji and martial skills to a more spontaneous situation.

Is Breathing Done Differently for Martial Purposes?

Some teachers tell their students that women will naturally use what is called in English "reverse breathing" (i.e., contract the abdomen/lower dantian when inhaling and expand the abdomen when inhaling) all the time, as it is natural to their gender. Conversely, the natural breathing mentioned in earlier chapters is normally said to be the required method for both sexes when doing qigong for health as well as slow form. This requires expanding while inhaling and contracting gently while exhaling.

As to martial training, most teachers tell students to exhale while striking and inhale while doing a lifting action, as in pushing. It's often taught in the internal arts in the context of reverse breathing, but others teach the opposite: You "fill out" the torso with an inhale as the ribcage and the abdomen open/expand.

While it is often said that you must consciously train in contracting the lower torso when inhaling and expanding it when exhaling, I personally don't practice conscious reverse breathing except in specific exercises and only for a limited number of repetitions. I do agree with those experts who say that natural abdominal breathing (relax/inhale the lower dantian, compress/exhale the lower dantian) is the most suitable way of breathing for standing qigong for health.

And I no longer have to pay any conscious attention to how I breathe while doing forms or being hit by my students—my body has learned how to adjust to those situations without my interference. In the same way, long-distance runners learn to breathe naturally and properly through gradually increasing how far they go and adjusting their pace to suit the rhythms of the breath. You can't run and pay attention to each inhalation or exhalation unless you want to ruin the competent job that your body will do automatically, if you are patient and train regularly and moderately.

Isn't one of your overall goals in taijiquan to let your body move naturally? With time and proper training, the end result seems to be that the entire torso learns to move with the breath like an accordion or old-style furnace bellows as it opens and closes, folds and unfolds, and that it can do this effectively and automatically when you are struck or pushed.

Martially, as with standing qigong and the long, slow form, the worst practice is holding the breath, as this causes the reactions to slow down, causes mental anxiety, and hardly makes it likely that you will be able to respond physically in a competent manner to training with a partner—much less dealing with a real aggressor!

Shouldn't Taijiquan Be Called Taijizhang?

You may remember from an earlier chapter that "quan" is usually translated as "fist" in English, although the Chinese character has less to do with clenching your hand than it does with symbolizing a skillful use of the hands. By contrast "zhang" is usually translated into English as "palm." Since most of the martial techniques in the Yang style involve an open hand, and not a fist, one might wonder why it's not called taijizhang. However, beginners normally find it easier to make a fist than to get the open hand to be relaxed enough to use, but not so "soft" that it gets hurt when making contact.

In most modern interpretations of the Yang style, a closed fist is used infrequently and, when this happens, the hand is folded into a fist shape in which the thumb is wrapped around the first two fingers when the hand is closed. There is less pressure in the last two fingers of the closed hand, as those digits will fold into the palm excessively if too much tension is present. The goal is to make a flat surface with the four fingers when curled and to strike with the last three fingers primarily, rather than with the big knuckles of the index and middle fingers.

A few older versions of the Yang style, including the one that I practice and teach from Erle Montaigue, uses a fist in which there is relatively little muscle tension except in the thumb and first finger. The tip of the thumb actually rests on the top of the closed first finger. The idea of this is to have both yang (the thumb and index finger are held relatively tightly) and yin (the other three fingers are held relatively loosely) in the hand with the yin aspect being somewhat predominant. In practical terms, the hand is more relaxed and has more potential for martial usage.

Using this kind of fist is very difficult to learn but has more versatility to its martial usage, as the tip of the thumb joint can also be used at odd angles against soft tissue targets. In addition, using this shape allows the wrist to settle properly when striking.

I'll add that practicing the various applications and training methods—with different levels of resistance from a partner—will start the process of conditioning the hands in terms of martial usage. This kind of training is not the same thing as banging your forearms or hands repeatedly (with or without herbal formulae) on various surfaces to toughen them. The latter is not normally considered an aspect of traditional Yang style. I don't have enough technical knowledge or experience in most of the other family styles to hazard a guess as to their current and past curricula.

Punching in the old forms is usually aimed at the heart rather than at the head as, in the old days, the students were told that striking the sternum above the area of the heart area crushed the "emotional mind," which resided in the middle dantian area of the chest. (Of course, any blow to this area can have quite a physical effect as well.)

It is also true that punching the head was not commonly recommended, as the head is a hard target to hit in all ways. All your opponent has to do is duck his head a few inches and you will be hitting the skull if you aim at the nose or eyes so that the danger of damaging the hand becomes very real. The other major consideration is avoiding accidentally hitting your closed fist on the opponent's elbows when he covers his ribs by pumping his relaxed elbows downward if the sides of the trunk are threatened. It might be wise to remember that Western boxers wrap their hands and wear gloves as much to protect their own hands and wrists as for any issue of making the impact safer for the other fighter.

On the other hand, if you practice open-hand strikes regularly, they will become as natural as closed-fist strikes and you are less likely to break your hand bones if you hit a bony target by mistake.

It can be instructive to look at the old internal styles and the structure of striking weapons. One of the details of hand-shape that becomes critical in making palm strikes or pushes as a practitioner matures is keeping the tiger mouth (the space between the thumb and first finger) slightly stretched and the first two fingers relatively yang to the last two fingers of each hand—particularly the "active" or "lead" hand in each posture.

Of course, if your middle finger is too stiff, the best you will achieve is a rude salute, but if your fingers are too soft and folded at all the joints, then you will only achieve a false sense of relaxation. Finding the "beautiful lady hand" in each posture is crucial to understanding the highest expressions of both martial and self-healing energy.

Another problem with learning the basic martial usage of the hands is the natural tendency to confine your practicing to striking the air while doing forms or practicing individual methods by yourself or with little or no contact on a training partner. Unfortunately, it is impossible, not just difficult, to learn how to efficiently and safely strike with the open hands if you don't practice making contact with a target of some kind—whether that target is a focus mitt, a padded shield, a heavy bag or makiwara, or a training partner wearing body armor so that he or she can safely be struck. In fact, all of these also create a natural progression in terms of learning how to use greater and greater amounts of power in your palm strikes while also maintaining the integrity of the various methods themselves.

A traditional way of practicing striking was to practice on a tree trunk (padded or otherwise) or on a heavy pole that had been sunk into the earth for that purpose. Even in North America, you can sometimes see older Chinese doing versions of this kind of training in parks early in the morning on suitable trees.

By the way, pulling your hand or foot technique just short of the target is not a good idea, as the neuromuscular system has cellular memory which allows it to remember the biological triggers learned from endlessly repeating the various movements you practice. If you always pull your strike just short of its target when you train or don't aim at the right target because you feel it's too dangerous for your training partner, then it's likely that you would not strike with power or accuracy if you used the same technique in a self-defense situation. Under stress, we usually do what we have trained to do. It should be obvious, but it isn't.

It is also important to remember that how hard and how well you can hit ultimately depends on how well you can reposition your body in relation to the opponent just before striking him or her. This use of timing and distancing is very difficult to learn if you only practice by yourself or with compliant partners and tends to take the longest to learn unless you are born with considerable aptitude for such martial attributes.

Let me put it simply: You may be able to strike like a battering ram or with the force of a whip, but if you can't get within the correct range to do so without being "blown out of the water" by the other fellow, then your palm-striking ability won't do you much good.

In other words, striking properly is one factor among many that has to be trained and fall into place before you can be as effective a martial artist as your potential allows.

Why the Obsession with Pushing in the Yang Style?

There seems to be an obsession among some modern Yang-style practitioners in terms of interpreting everything done with the open-hand as being a push rather than a strike. There may have been some truth in this originally, as I have been told more than once by Chen stylists that this preference for what looks like pushing, tripping, and grappling goes back to the origins of the art in the late 19th century when its adherents had to deal with opponents who might be wearing armor of some kind. It certainly makes more sense to knock someone down or attack his joints to disarm or control him than to punch a helmet or breastplate.

However, the Yang style was created much later than the Chen style (which is noted almost as much for its use of the elbows as it is noted for pushing) and the use of armor was no longer a factor in determining tactics in combat, thanks to the increasing use of firearms on the Chinese mainland. Although a good practitioner would still have been forced to have some understanding of wrestling, grappling, and joint-locking simply because of the prevalence of those kinds of methods in many of the older Chinese martial arts, it is also true that the most important aspect of pushing can only come through the concept of what I call the principle of *push and pull,* which is usually explained in older writings as being like the action of sawing wood. Even in today's technological world, most of us will have some idea of how to use a manual hand saw, in that the blade must apply even pressure, the edge of the tool must be properly sharpened, and the drawback is integral to cutting smoothly in that one direction sets up the other for maximum speed and efficiency in the cutting process.

It is also true that a good woodworker will learn, through trial and error, to hold the saw firmly but without tension, will use his arm and subtle movements of the body to power the arm holding and controlling the tool. He or she won't just push indiscriminately with a tight grip and a frantic use of the shoulder muscles—well, not for long, anyway!

However, this analogy isn't quite precise enough, as the originators of taiji were referring more precisely to the use of a two-person saw. Chain saws have made this piece of apparatus obsolete in North America at least, so it is rare to find such tools unless they are antiques hanging on walls or being used in lumberjack competitions. For those who have never seen a two-person saw, it has a long, thick, and heavy blade with a sawing edge on one (sometimes both) sides. It was used before power tools to saw tree trunks into crude planks and has a handle at each end so that it can be wielded by two people instead of one.

Those who are familiar with the shifting patterns in most two-person push-hands methods will understand that it mimics in some ways the actions of two people cooperating to saw through wood with such an implement. One person applies force in a pushing action while the other must draw or "pull" from his end to amplify the speed and power of the other person. If one worker is out in his or her timing, then the blade won't cut efficiently or will actually bind and stop within the cut.

In martial terms, one player practices listening and drawing skills while the other practices listening and pushing skills. The first level of push-hands skill is learning how to coordinate this to-and-fro without losing contact and without having it become a meaningless choreography. As in all aspects of push-hands training, the most difficult thing is to pay attention properly even when doing choreographed movement.

In self-defense terms, push and pull as a concept implies that you have learned to do this action so sensitively and so smoothly that, if your attacker binds up and resists your actions, you can change direction suddenly to pull him when he resists your push and vice-versa. Learning how to do this against an opponent who offers some resistance and has skill as well is not an easy thing and forms the essence of the strategy of any close-contact martial art. The photos on the interaction between play the lute and brush knee in the section on posture applications in Chapter 5 illustrate one martial aspect of this.

In the end, a good push can be a very useful martial tool if you do so with the whole body and not just with the arms or chest. A good push can be "percussive" and shake or jar the person being pushed in that manner, leaving them stunned and vulnerable to follow-up techniques. A good push can uproot and imbalance or topple an unstable opponent. A good push can send someone flying and twisting either upward or downward. Pushing properly also involves having one of your feet between his feet and under his center of gravity, or hooked around one of his feet or on top of his toes as he gets launched.

Pushing is less useful if that is all you can do and you don't survive getting close enough to do it. The obsession with both rooting and pushing in many of the modern versions of taiji is ridiculous from a practical self-defense perspective.

On the other hand, It is also important to consider historically that it was a crime punishable by death in old China to kill someone—even if you did so in self-defense. So there might well have been a tendency to use less immediately lethal reactions by at least some of the practitioners of taiji, especially when the art came to Beijing and the other large cities where, one would assume, the rule of law would have been more strictly enforced than in a rural village or small town.

Finally, pushing can be somewhat safer for the students than striking or throwing and I agree with those authorities who feel that the apparent emphasis on "pushing" in modern push-hands came about primarily to make some of the training methods a little safer for daily practice. I am also told that practicing with strangers in a park in China or another city can certainly bring a quick appreciation of just how "martial" a good push can be as you go flying into a garbage can or pond. I have also done it and seen it used with spectacular results when a little too much "lift" is used and your partner hits the wall harder than either of you wanted.

Unfortunately, many modern teachers don't have enough of a martial base of any kind to be able to understand just how useful a push can be—and how limiting it can be if that is all you can do in combative terms.

What is Investing in Loss?

The late Cheng Man Ching is reported, by some sources, to have exhorted his students often to "invest in loss," which can be understood in a variety of ways depending on your experience with taiji and the internal arts.

I like to suggest to my students that they think of this as being advice to learn from your mistakes rather than get mad at yourself or your training partner over not learning everything the easy way or immediately. Particularly when it comes to being pushed around or struck, even when the injury is more to your dignity than your body, the tendency is to get mad and overreact or to give up such training prematurely.

In this regard, it is particularly important when practicing with a partner to refrain from getting angry with him if he seems to keep "besting" you during such training. Learn from your mistakes rather than just blaming your partner or getting irritated with yourself. In addition, don't avoid practicing with someone just because you find them a less desirable partner for whatever reason—it's good training in patience and perseverance to work with those you like less. On the other hand, a good teacher will not encourage or put up with bullying in any form.

Even with the more gentle expressions of basic training, like sensitivity drills, the temptation is first to refuse to acknowledge that you have made a mistake, then to look for someone else to blame, and then finally to come up with an excuse for why you failed. For example, your partner knocks you off-balance and your first reply is "No, I didn't move my feet," when you finally admit that you did lose your balance, then the next reaction is often, "My partner used too much force!" and the last bit of ego-defense is likely to be, "Well, I wasn't ready!"

Being overly defensive is hardly unique to push-hands or learning form, but it certainly shows up frequently in those endeavors. The first step is to recognize that there are things that you need to work on in yourself that are hindering your progress. Seems like common sense, but it's amazing how many students have trouble identifying their problem areas. Sometimes they can't see the problems; quite often they do but refuse to acknowledge their existence.

In this regard, I remember the end of an introductory session on slow form that I had done with a group of potential students. One lady came up to me afterward and announced, as she walked out the door, that she would not be coming back to class, as she wasn't paying me to correct her constantly! Better students realize that this is exactly what they are paying me for until they develop the ability to correct themselves.

Now, investing in loss is hard enough in solo work or in the rarefied atmosphere of a modern push-hands class in which slow-motion and sensitivity are the key words and a roomful of middle-class people of all ages look as if they are engaging in vertical foreplay in slow-motion.

It gets harder still when someone is repeatedly beating his way through your defenses, punching you or pushing you vigorously into a wall. In this case, it is almost impossible to rationalize your weaknesses—you either learn from them, refuse to return to that kind of training environment, or lose your temper and escalate the training to the level of, "Oh, yeah? Take this!"

All are counterproductive. In the end, keeping your eyes open and your mind attentive to what your are trying to absorb are essential learning tools, as is "investing in loss."

Separating Fact from Fantasy

After many years of training and seeing a variety of Chinese martial arts experts in action, I have not seen any convincing evidence that the so-called "empty force" (kong jing), the ability to project qi from a distance to negatively affect an aggressor, is anything other than an "empty farce" in martial terms.

It is true that projecting qi for healing purposes is considered legitimate by some traditionalists. However, it is generally considered, even by these, that it is only useful at very close quarters and only by an exceptionally skillful and experienced qigong doctor.

Those few martial experts who talk about affecting someone's energy field in a martial context will again say that close proximity is essential, and only as a way of weakening the other person's energy field to make him more vulnerable to the actual strikes that follow immediately. In other words, such knowledge is relatively useless unless you know how to fight and can keep the attacker from harming you without such specialized knowledge.

To make it even more confusing, when a proponent of empty force is asked for a demonstration on someone other than one of his students, he or she will often say that it is too dangerous to do this on someone who hasn't had special training. If the demonstration goes ahead anyway and the master fails, he or she will often say that it failed because the subject's qi was too strong.

A common reaction when a demonstration of qi power fails is for the "master" to ask if you do martial arts and then say, "Oh, your qi must be strong because of your training." Other great rationalizations I have heard are, "I only demonstrate on my students because they have done the necessary training to make them immune to my power" and "I won't demonstrate on you because my qi is so strong that I might rip off your muscles if I touched your arm."

On a traditional martial level, those who told the young Chinese patriot boxers at the turn of the 20th century that their paper charms and esoteric qigong practices would stop the bullets of the foreign "devils" during the Boxer Rebellion were probably not all trying to mislead their followers. Most probably sincerely believed in what they were saying or had experienced the ability of the mind to minimize injury and stop pain and bleeding from a variety of minor wounds. Faith, in this case, was the cause of death and injury.

However, it is almost criminal to teach modern beginners with no martial experience that they can put all of their trust in "making a golden bell cover for the torso" out of weiqi or of not having to bother to learn physically how to defend themselves because they can learn to project qi at an attacker. In some cases, the instructor actually begins to believe that they have some mystical ability because the techniques seem to work on some of their students or cooperative peers.

However, as in most matters, it is not a cut-and-dried proposition to decide who is a complete charlatan as opposed to who has skill mixed with a traditional approach to the use of energy. For example, some years ago I purchased a videotaped demonstration by an elderly Yang-style taiji master based in Southeast Asia. This teacher (now dead) had a very good reputation as a fighter when younger, as well as a teacher with decades of experience. As the cassette that I had purchased was in a different video format than I could use, I had to pay to have it converted into the appropriate format at a local business that did such work.

When I returned to get it, the middle-aged fellow who ran that business handed me the tapes and blurted out as I paid, "Sir, you are wasting your money. I watched this pushing stuff and it is all BULLSHIT. My son is a black belt in tae kwon do and I know what fightings [sic] is all about."

And then he pointed to the Chinese businessman sitting in the corner waiting his turn and added, "He watched it with me; we both saw these grown men throwing themselves about from silly pushes."

I looked at the Chinese fellow, who nodded his head politely and said in heavily accented English "Taiji, very good. Make you healthy—not for fighting."

Well, after I watched the tape at home I had to acknowledge why those two could have jumped to such conclusions. The old master was very fluid, despite his age, but there were also too many instances of his touching a student who would then fall down or sometimes roll backward several times and off the stage. It's too bad, because some of the senior students who demonstrated were very fluid and I liked the forms shown in many ways. Furthermore, some of the senior students who demonstrated had real "looseness" and skill and I always take that as a good sign when at least some of a teacher's students develop along similar lines.

The old master himself also had obvious martial skill, which makes it even sadder when the demonstrations by adoring students become ridiculous from a common sense point of view. As to the students hurling themselves backward off the stage, such nonsense won't impress anyone with a lot of fighting experience, but it will fool those people who are unable or unwilling to train more effectively.

I think the idea of being able to defend yourself at a distance is very seductive to the types of students often attracted to taijiquan and the internal arts, until they find out that hard work, sweat, and the odd bruise are the main secrets to learning how to defend yourself in the first few years at least. Most of these leave the legitimate instructors to go in search of those teachers who specialize in mystery, neo-Daoism, and what a cynic might call "stage magic."

This seems to be particularly prevalent in qigong practices in recent years. There was an American television evangelist, as well as a famous long-distance Chinese qigong healer, in the United States who used to get people to touch the television screen so that their palms would seem to be in contact with the quack's palm held up to the camera. When people felt the static discharge of the screen into their hands at home, it was really healing power being transmitted!

We had one young Chinese lady locally who taught women's self-defense classes in which she taught them to punch with their thumbs wrapped inside the fingers, as this made their hands "packed with qi." Human nature being what it is, I would imagine that many of her students blamed their resultant injuries on not having done it well enough or not having enough qi.

The problem for these self-deceivers lies in working only with their own students, or in growing to believe that they have some mystical power because they can impress lesser-skilled people in a controlled situation like a workshop.

But it can be risky to call such "masters" out, as some do have enough fighting skill to be dangerous if they think you are trying to embarrass them. So be prepared for them to use unnecessary force in their supposed "light touch" knockouts if you're the dummy in their demonstration. I know, first hand, of one idiot who broke a workshop attendee's arm in an effort to demonstrate his supposed light touch strike to cause knockout—to the horror of the dojo owner who had sponsored the workshop.

I also think that many of these hype-masters do actually start to believe their own stories after having repeated them often enough to audiences that swallow the stories or have never seen better. It is easy on many levels to be a "big fish in a small pond" if the people we teach have never seen the ocean and sharks. And a lie repeated often enough begins to sound like the truth, even to the ears of the deceiver.

On the other hand, I think that anyone who has been involved in the internal martial arts long enough has witnessed or experienced "a few weird events." I have witnessed stuff that I still can't explain fully, but that doesn't mean that I am willing to suspend my common sense or try to fool my students into believing that I have extraordinary martial and healing powers by using sleight-of-hand skills.

I agree that it is important to keep an open mind, but I also would have more respect for those who claim such esoteric skills if they could demonstrate them on noncompliant subjects with objective observers to record the event.

Isn't that the best part of Western science, that it asks us to question everything and not to assume that something is true simply because we want to believe it is so?

DIM MAK

Tsien hueh (as dim mak is often called) refers to the martial use of the acupuncture points to cause temporary or permanent damage to the qi flow in the meridians and certain acupuncture points, as well as to the organs and nervous system of the body. It is an ugly but fascinating aspect of learning taijiquan and can be considered the yang to the yin, or healing use, of those same points.

On a pragmatic level, the value of striking, twisting, or sealing these points often lies in affecting arterial blood flow, dislocating bones, tearing muscles and ligaments, or traumatizing major nerves. An experienced practitioner can hope to do this only if he or she has a profound understanding of fighting strategy as well as a detailed knowledge of point location and manipulation. There are over 360 points on the acupuncture meridians that are commonly used for healing purposes, and just over a hundred that are considered to be particularly useful in martial terms.

In recent years, a number of reputable books that talk about the existence of these dim mak skills in early taiji, including those by Erle Montaigue, have been published in English. Chinese sources also mention this. For example, the existence of such "secret" training is mentioned in *Lost T'ai Chi Classics From the Late Ching Dynasty* as translated by Douglas Wile (State University of New York Press, 1996) in Chapter 37 of a thought-to-be-lost text called *Yang Family Forty Chapters*. The title of that chapter is *"Oral Transmission of the Theory of Life and Death Acupoints."*

It is also essential to consider the psychological aspect of such training. If you're convinced that an expert in dim mak can knock you out with a relatively light strike to your forearm, or that your heart will stop if points just above your elbow are squeezed forcefully, then it would be surprising if you didn't feel a little nervous when hit or squeezed on those points. In the old days, if you were a dim mak expert and everyone knew about it, then you were less likely to be attacked (except by another expert, who would presumably have developed the skills necessary to counteract yours). However, if you struck a non-expert, then he or she would expect to develop severe side effects even if you hadn't done any real physical harm—and probably would due to the power of suggestion. It is also equally true that a confident fighter who did not know of your reputation would probably not be the least intimidated if you simply squeezed or struck those same points.

In any case, I am convinced that the dim mak works, even if only in the sense that the most useful points are often over nerve centers or arteries or organs that are particularly sensitive to pressure, like the kidneys or liver. I also agree with Erle that such skills, while a legitimate heritage of the Yang style, are not easy to understand, even on a theoretical level. In this regard, knowing the locations of a few such points on the human body and their theoretical usage will only get you beaten to a pulp unless you can already defend yourself adequately without such skills.

Having said this, I also think that there may well be more to this than meets the eye, at least on rare occasion. Erle Montaigue talks about dim mak really only being effective when you "put in the evil qi" and I used to think that such talk was nonsense. Now, after having met him and a few other experts, I'm not so sure. On the other hand, those who seem convincing in such talk also have the physical and fighting skills to make such tactics work—even without the application of qi, evil or otherwise.

While such martial skills may have been necessary when created in lawless feudal times, they have little place in modern life. I also think that in the long run it is better to learn the healing use of these points through acupressure or tuina or shiatsu-style massage. The refined use of qi in the internal arts, no matter how you define and explore such knowledge, should promote good health, not destroy it.

Although he is often unfairly branded as a martial eccentric for his views on traditional dim mak, Erle Montaigue, unlike many of those who have done workshop tours and produced videos or books on this subject, has gone out of his way to help debunk the myths and demonstrate how important it is to avoiding practicing such tactics in a haphazard or incredulous manner.

Oh, and by the way, I know that some of these points work well because he has knocked me out with them. There aren't many that I would voluntarily be a guinea pig for in such demonstrations, but Erle really is one in a million.

IS MARTIAL CROSS-TRAINING REALLY A GOOD IDEA?

Cross-training can be interpreted in two ways: doing supplementary strengthening or stretching methods other than those taught by your teacher, or learning and practicing another martial system. It used to be fairly common for taijiquan teachers of any style to discourage their students from training elsewhere—whether with another Yang-style teacher or in a completely different martial art. This attitude is still occasionally encountered and can be grossly exaggerated to the point where students are told not to read books about other interpretations of taiji or practice other forms of exercise (i.e., yoga, weight-training), or are asked to sign waivers promising that they won't study elsewhere while taking classes.

There were, of course, always exceptions to this generalization and one of the most common in the Chinese internal arts was students being encouraged to cross-train in both xingyiquan and baguazhang, or in one or both of those with taijiquan. However, those doing this were usually quite skillful in one system before starting to study the other. This was considered preferable to studying with two teachers at the same time, as this could be both confusing for the student as well as show a lack of loyalty to both the teachers involved.

In practical terms, if you are doing or learning another martial art at the same time as you start learning the Yang style, you will find that time is inelastic and that it can be difficult to schedule enough time to do justice to more than one system at a time. Still, we can all fall prey to the urge to try something new, hence the temptation to learn solo form after form (without ever mastering any) or of regularly switching from martial or exercise style to style every few months.

After many years of training, I now have some understanding of the words of one of my former teachers, who said that good students will get a taste of whatever systems they can, partly to understand how the common principles of these arts can be legitimately interpreted in very different ways on a physical level, and partly to improve their understanding of their main disciplines. It also allows the serious student the opportunity to decide if he or she should switch styles as his or her main focus.

It also doesn't hurt to have access to scientific approaches to strengthening the body in terms of cardiovascular and weight training, not to mention stretching, that actually is in accordance with the modern understanding of how the body functions optimally. Many of the stretches and strengthening methods of the traditional versions of taijiquan and the martial arts in general are more than a little suspect as to their being good for the long-term health of practitioners. Older is not always better when it comes to physical training.

Another valid reason for cross-training is to fill in the gaps in your understanding of the four basic martial approaches to using the body: kicking for long-range, punching for intermediate range, and wrestling and joint-locking for grappling range. In some ways, you can think of wrestling as being designed to deal with kicking and punching, while joint-locking is a method of both supporting and countering grappling skills. Kicking and punching are used against each other and to support the functional usage of the grappling range methods. Very few modern styles or teachers will do more than focus on one or two of these ranges/methods in their own practice or teaching.

One aspect of the Chinese martial arts that has always made me a little grumpy is the tendency for instructors to imply or say that they are masters of all four methods and many distinct styles. It is not uncommon to meet someone whose business card or flyers list him or her as a master of wing chun, shaolin, both Chen and Yang taiji, xingyiquan, and baguazhang as well as qigong of different types—and maybe some karate and tae kwon do as well.

Sadly, most modern practitioners don't have a solid foundation before they go off studying other approaches and lack the aptitude to absorb not only the similarities, but the differences between the arts that they are learning. Usually the students who are most keen to cross-train prematurely tend to focus on how the new art(s) are similar to what they already know as opposed to trying to analyze how the new system or teacher does things differently. And, as sometimes the differences are subtle, it can be problematic to "sort the wheat from the chaff." Of course, I could be wrong. (My wife assures me that this is often the case.)

I have met a few teachers and practitioners over the years who actually are good at a variety of arts, but these are rare exceptions. The average martial generalist of this kind is only fooling himself or his students by teaching one or two main styles and then a smattering of forms or methods from the other arts.

It is essential to remember that there is little benefit from simply learning a form or training method from one style and then believing that you somehow understood the entire system of which that solo form can only be a very small part!

It's quite depressing to surf the 'Net and see Web site after Web site promoting these schools and new styles to the general martial public. While I'm sure that some of these innovators are doing their best and may even have something to offer to beginners, I'm equally sure that even more are fooling only themselves and/or their own students with their abilities, or are creating a new style to make money or boost their egos.

I do believe that any competent teacher will encourage any experienced student to research other martial and exercise systems, at least for a period of time and from a variety of sources. However, for beginners, the issue is a little more complicated.

Beginners

Although I don't insist that new students immediately stop training in any other martial discipline that they may have mastered in order to learn from me, they may well eventually reach a point at which they must choose the path that best suits them at that point in their lives. Human nature is such that the average beginner usually resists or resents this need to "start over" completely. I have been faced with such a situation several times over the decades and it is never an easy decision on any level.

In my experience, it's difficult to say which is better: having a beginner who is experienced martially, or who has no such experience. In particular, those with hard-style experience can be either the best or the worst of students, although at least they are already used to some physical contact and have a level of fitness that is often lacking in older beginners coming from the modern qigong or taiji traditions.

For the More Experienced

Cross-training can also mean studying the various aspects of close combat (striking versus kicking, grappling versus standup, etc.), as most modern variations of the fighting arts will specialize both in stylistic terms and according to the preferences of each teacher within those systems.

You can't really appreciate the difference by reading books on the subjects—although you wouldn't know that from many of the discussions that take place on Internet discussion forums. Martial geniuses can mobilize and use effectively all of these forms of strategy. The average expert understands one strategy really well and has learned some effective methods to counter someone trying the other strategies against him. The average student has no idea what I am talking about.

In terms of self-defense skills, I would put my money on an experienced Western boxer (even an older, out-of-shape exponent) who has to fight any type of modern martial artist, black belt or not. Boxing has had its ups and downs over the decades, but the "sweet science" is just as profound in its principles and techniques as any of the other martial arts when it is well-taught and practiced. It has the advantage of simplicity and its only disadvantages are that the stamina and conditioning required to fight competitively—even at an amateur level—make it only a young man's art.

Years ago I was friends with a 50-year-old man who was learning taiji "for fun." Kenny had been an amateur and professional boxer and still trained and coached young boxers. It was both funny and sad to see him flatten the younger and fitter taiji instructors who sparred with him at the school where we trained. Anyone who says an experienced boxer is automatically inferior to a traditional martial artist in combative terms has never had the experience of meeting someone like my old friend.

Particularly for those interested in the Yang style as a self-defense system, I think that it is important to learn the basics of both standup and ground fighting in the early stages of training. In particular, this means having learned how to do a fall and roll safely on a variety of surfaces.

I was fortunate that one of my best teachers, Allan Weiss, had a strong background in throwing arts before taking up taiji. He insisted that all of his students learn the basics of such techniques. His classes were held for many years in an aikido dojo, so we had the use of tatami matting to learn these essential martial skills.

In the end, if you study one art deeply, you will learn a great deal, but you also limit your potential for growth by not studying how other systems do the same thing slightly (or greatly) differently. Conversely, if you spend a year in one system and move on to another, try to learn several systems at the same time, or dabble in workshops with an endless list of instructors, you can gain a superficial veneer of skill but may never actually have learned anything in depth.

True experiential learning of any mind/body discipline is first a process of accumulation and then a process of de-cluttering, simplification, and specialization.

CULTURAL ISSUES

Do You Have to be Fluent in Chinese?

I don't speak or read Chinese and for many years didn't think that it mattered in terms of doing a decent interpretation of taijiquan. Now I'm not so sure anymore. As I mentioned in an earlier chapter, part of the problem for North American students lies in their immigrant teachers having little or no English language skills in terms of explaining the finer details of practice to their native-born students, or being able to answer questions in a second language.

Having someone who translates the expert's words isn't always a blessing, either, as this kind of communication can be cumbersome and doesn't always succeed on a technical level when the translator isn't both a good linguist and a good taiji practitioner.

I remember an incident in the early days of my taiji study in which one of my fellow students was trying to ask one of our teachers for his opinion on her back troubles. The late Mr. Choi (a wonderful human being and teacher) was a fairly recent arrival from Hong Kong and his English tended to fail him outside of a few basic situations. However, the woman student in question knew that he was a skillful TCM doctor and wanted his advice on the chronic pain she suffered due to an old injury. Mr. Choi was still smiling politely as he listened to her repeating her question for the third time, but he finally motioned for one of the Chinese students to come over. The latter spoke excellent English but was a little scattered as a human being. Mr. Choi spoke to him in Chinese and gestured at the woman who was talking to him. The Chinese student listened respectfully and then turned to the young woman. "Teacher would like to know what your problem is due to?" The woman smiled, grateful that she would finally be understood, and said, "Please tell Mr. Choi that I hurt my back some time ago in a car crash and it has never been the same afterward. I was wondering if he could have a look at it for me to give me his opinion."

The Chinese student nodded and said, "No problem." Then he turned to Mr. Choi and repeated her words to our teacher almost verbatim, but *in English*. Those of us watching had difficulty restraining our laughter, but the principals didn't seem to realize what had happened at first and then switched to Mandarin.

Many years after that incident, I still don't think that you need to be able to read the classics in their original language to be able to do good Yang taiji, but I have also come to realize that the finer details of practice are often obscured because of language difficulties while in class or through questionable translations of the surviving texts that have become known collectively as the taiji classics. Even a good modern Chinese translator may not understand the context of words that were written 50 or 100 years ago. As I pointed out in an earlier chapter, the old texts were often written in note form for experienced students, not as primers for beginners or the uninitiated.

For example, sung is commonly translated into English as "relax," although in Chinese it has more complex meanings and really implies that one is comfortable within one's structure and movements. Part of the training of taijiquan is devoted to learning how to do this while avoiding extremes of either constant tension or constant limpness. In this context, a martial translation of sung has more to do with "springiness" or "elasticity" and can be likened to the flexible resilience of bamboo.

I would assume that the first English-language translators were not taiji experts, as there weren't any non-Chinese experts in the 1960s in North America to do such work when the first English-language taiji books appeared. Their translations stuck and became common usage. Several of my friends earn their livings as translators and it is obvious from their comments and stories that translating any technical language in and out of English is a challenging task.

Particularly when the translator doesn't know much about the technical or cultural side of whatever they are translating, being accurate to the original can be a daunting task. I would assume that translators themselves often resort to consulting an existing translation to help them with a new project. So, for example, if the translator sees "pull" in one or two existing translations and doesn't happen to be a taiji expert, he or she will probably translate "cai" as "pull" instead of "pluck" in the new text—thus helping unwittingly to perpetuate the poor translation.

Finally, human beings are creatures of habit and inertia is a driving factor (pun intended!) in how we approach things. For example, the modern keyboard is essentially the same as it was decades ago when it was designed to SLOW typing speeds, so that the old metal hammers holding the individual characters didn't jam together if someone typed too quickly and efficiently. Even though more efficient keyboards have been created in recent years, inertia has guaranteed that the old one is still in use as people are reluctant to switch from the familiar to the unfamiliar. So it is with translations of the old terms.

In the end, a few modern North American experts will have a real advantage in understanding both their instructors and the old writings, because of their language skills in both English and Chinese as well as their martial skills. The rest of us will have to struggle along with translations to the best of our ability.

SHOULD YOU STUDY IN CHINA OR THE ORIENT TO REALLY LEARN TAIJI?

I have never actually had the urge to go to China or Taiwan to study taijiquan there. That is partly because I was able to find decent enough teachers in North America who spoke my language, and partly because I have heard mixed reports over the years that I have been training from those who did spend time learning taijiquan or other Chinese martial systems in the Far East.

China has become a world power in recent years. What can you say about a country of over a billion people whose current government is almost schizophrenic in its attempts to control this huge population, while still allowing the growth of what is essentially a free-market economy that has made this country one of the most powerful on Earth? Well, in terms of taiji training, what you can say is that many Chinese teachers have discovered that there is a great deal of hard currency to be made from catering to North American and European students.

Open any relevant magazine and you will easily find ads from teachers who are organizing jaunts overseas. These are sight-seeing expeditions that also offer the chance to spend a few days, a few weeks, or a few months studying in Chen Village or at a Chinese Martial Sports College, or even at a newly rebuilt Daoist monastery—complete with restaurant and souvenir shops on Mount Wudang.

There are also many teachers in North America with links to teachers in China who are all too happy to organize—for a price—your visit to study with their teacher, or who arrange workshop tours of those masters in North America on a regular basis. As with anything, these are sometimes excellent opportunities for serious practitioners to boost their skill levels by learning in the country of origin of their art, and sometimes it is just another rip-off that finds the student home sooner than he or she expected, with intestinal parasites and financially poorer though not much wiser about taiji—but perhaps a whole lot wiser about human nature in other countries.

I am also told that it is difficult to learn real martial arts away from the taiji tourist traps unless you have a letter of introduction to a good teacher and you stay long enough to build some trust with that teacher, assuming that he or she accepts you in his or her classes in the first place. And remember the language issue? I am also told that you shouldn't bother going unless you have a talent for picking up languages or already have some Chinese under your belt.

Many current teachers in North America have made the pilgrimage for shorter or longer periods of time and done serious study with serious teachers in Taiwan or on the mainland. Unfortunately, for every Tim Cartmell, Andrea Falk, or Sam Masich who has lived in China or traveled regularly to train with teachers, there are dozens of others who have spent a weekend or a week with someone who was all too happy to have their photos taken with a well-paying foreigner, or to give him or her some meaningless certificates of attendance.

I have even heard that it is sometimes considered a source of pride to have the most foreign dilettante students in your fold among the teachers in places like Beijing, where they get a lot of foreign taiji tourists.

It is also worth knowing that many Chinese practitioners are rather anxious to put foreigners "in their place" when training with them and it is wise to have very good skills in the first place, or to show a little deference when engaged in push-hands and the martial training.

There are no New-Age practitioners in the hotbeds of taiji in the Chinese parks. You will be sent flying if you can't keep up to the pace or if you show a lack of respect for the originators of the art.

Do You Have to Study Daoism to Learn Taijiquan?

As with being fluent in Chinese, understanding any Chinese belief system (e.g., Daoism, Confucianism, Buddhism), even if it is only on a superficial intellectual level, is a lot like taking your grandmother's chicken soup when you have the flu—it can't hurt.

For those with strong religious feelings, there is no need to embrace any foreign religion or system of thought to be a successful practitioner of any style of taijiquan. However, we do live in a more conservative age these days, and a surprising number of clerics seem to feel that their flock may be tainted spiritually by practicing taijiquan because of its connection to Chinese religion and philosophy.

More than once over the years I have read articles by fundamentalist Christians and Muslims denouncing the practice of taijiquan and qigong as being somehow the tools of Satan. It is sometimes a surprise for new students to find out that some of the modern Chinese leaders in the family styles of taijiquan are evangelical Christians of different denominations, and even occasionally Muslim, as there are large Muslim minorities in parts of China.

Many middle-class white exponents, however, will go to the opposite extreme and try to become more Chinese than the native practitioners of old! You don't have to wear an ancient outfit, learn to speak or read Mandarin or Cantonese, and spout "fortune-cookie" wisdom to benefit from your training—in fact, it is usually an impediment to progress.

On the other hand, Daoism can be relevant to those of us who study taiji on many levels. Zhang San Feng and a number of other semimythical Daoists have been given credit for creating the fundamental principles of taiji. Lao Zhi may be the most famous of the Daoist philosophers, but it is important to remember that the principles laid out in his marvelous little book the *Dao De Jing* were already an intrinsic part of Chinese culture at the time that the first editions were circulating among the literati of old China.

Acceptance, or "going with the flow," is integral to the Daoist experience, as is *wuwei* (noninterference). In terms of push-hands and the martial function, acceptance of the incoming force is essential if one to to redirect it as opposed to resisting it. In fact, acceptance is as central to being enlightened as it is to defending yourself. If you fight the idea of accepting the existence of an incoming blow or aggressor, it is likely to paralyze both your will to fight and your physical reactions.

Similarly, taiji practice can lead to embracing "accepting" in the sense that you let go of fear and of the psychological need to control and plan what will happen to you. The impossibility of controlling life is clearly demonstrated in microcosm by trying to plan ahead of time how you would cope with an aggressor's attacks. In this way, a self-defense application becomes a microcosm of dealing with psychological aggression in daily life, just as the human body and mind were seen by the Daoists as a microcosm of the universe and the forces at play within that universe.

Lao Zhi advises us to discard learning and desire and to cultivate stillness to find, in that stillness, movement. The sage who followed him, Chuang Zhi, wrote, "He who practices the Way does less and less every day, does less and goes on doing less until he reaches the point where he does nothing and yet there is nothing that remains undone."

In solo practice, the taiji practitioner begins solo form with stillness and returns to it after completing that flow of movement that is the form. With time and practice, he or she learns to shed the layers of intellectual, emotional, and muscular armor accumulated over the years in a vain attempt to control the uncontrollable—life.

In the combative side of taiji, the practitioner learns to be still on a mental level and to find that sense of "stillness" even when moving quickly to deal with an aggressor. This relates to the idea of having central equilibrium as the center of your understanding of the five directions.

Another Daoist attitude necessary for the understanding of taiji is the use of intuition as opposed to empirical knowledge. Rather than trying to memorize the right technique to use at the right moment, the experienced practitioner allows himself or herself to flow around and through the "cracks" between the incoming forces to dissipate them while counterattacking with whatever force is appropriate at the time.

Such intuition is best learned through the give-and-take of an apprenticeship with someone who has "got it" (or at least occasionally glimpsed it). Similarly, taiji, despite the proliferation of books—yes, even this one—as well as videos, cannot really be learned beyond a certain point except through a demanding teacher/student relationship.

The Daoist artist uses blank space and the most tentative of strokes to create images that seem, to the uninitiated, to be unfinished. In this way, like the best of modern expressionistic art, the viewer can add an element of his or her own imagination to complete what is shown on paper or ceramic. Such works of art are frustrating to the observer who needs a detailed structure to feel comfortable, but are magical to those who are willing to interpret the image from their own perspective as well as that of the artist.

In the same way, the eventual formlessness of fighting can be intimidating to those students who can only relate to the structure of prearranged training methods. Freestyle training becomes an exercise in futility for such students. On the other hand, some can relate well to formlessness but have a great deal of difficulty relating to and learning precision of posture as well the structured training methods.

A particularly appealing aspect of Daoism is its use of humor. The works of Lao Zhi and Chuang Zhi are filled with puns and humorous analogies. There is not the notion that things that are important must necessarily be serious. I would suspect that the best of the living Daoists are able to transmit this sense of laughter and of play even as they transmit the essence of their experience of life. Similarly, the best teachers of taiji take their art, but not themselves, too seriously and teach through humor and by demonstrating the love that they feel for their discipline.

To paraphrase an old expression, "You can lead a student to the Yang style but you can't make him or her drink!" You can only demonstrate how and why such training can be sustaining on many levels.

The best teachers do not encourage violence, but are also not afraid to make their martial practice realistic within the bounds of training safely. Lao Zhi did not write that war and violence must be avoided at all costs, but rather that they must not be glorified. In his words, "Victorious armies should be greeted with the rites of mourning for the lives they have been forced to take and not with rejoicing for the victory itself."

Daoism was a flower that grew from the mire of war and social disorder in the Period of the Warring States. When you consider just how stressful modern life is for many of us today, is it any wonder that the benevolent eccentricity of taiji and Daoism has new meaning for increasing numbers of people?

It is also difficult to avoid romanticizing and misunderstanding any aspect of old Chinese culture and some modern experts have written convincingly of the need to reevaluate the Western fascination with Daoism. One such text that is a good place to start this kind of research is *The Taoism of the Western Imagination and the Taoism of China: De-Colonializing the Exotic Teachings of the East,* which was presented by Russell Kirkland at the University of Tennessee on October 20th, 1997. You can access this text at several Web sites, including www.daoistcenter.org/Articles/Articles_pdf/Kirkland.pdf

As I get older, I find myself increasingly impatient with those who have rejected their own heritage in favor of alien cultures simply because they can't be bothered to be selective over what they embrace from the new and preserve from the old.

The Authenticity of the Taiji Classics

There is a collection of short texts written by early masters like Ly Yi Yu, Chen Wei Ming, and Yang Cheng-fu, among others, as well as others from an even earlier period like Wang Zhong Yue and Zhang San Feng. These short writings are often quoted and translated in many English books on taiji and given the authority that is usually granted to religious texts. Like some of the famous religious texts, their authenticity is somewhat suspect.

Closer to our time, it was common enough for texts to be ghostwritten in China. For example, it is generally accepted that Yang Cheng-fu was functionally illiterate, as were many of his generation, and that all three of the books attributed to him were actually written by three of his more literate disciples.

Reach even further back and some of the writings attributed to Chang San-feng and Yang Lu-chan were also more than likely written by practitioners who wanted to add a ring of authenticity to their efforts by attributing them to more prestigious sources. I suppose that it is one of the great ironies of taijiquan that at least some of the oldest such texts are likely forgeries in the sense that they were not written by the authors to which they are attributed.

An educated Chinese of that time would not have seen this as inappropriate, nor would he have found anything unusual in attributing the beginnings of a family style to a figure like Zhang San Feng who was, in many versions of the story, a supernatural figure. "The older, the better" was a Western saying that would have made much sense to a literate Chinese reader in those days.

As I have mentioned previously, it is also important to remember that many of the old masters created the lesser texts that have survived to this day for their senior students and not for outsiders or the general public. These were most often in the form of oral "songs" (a Westerner would call these poems) that were a shorthand way of remembering essential concepts and theory.

It seems strange to modern students who aren't old enough to remember having to do extensive memory work in school (it has sadly gone out of style in North America, at least) that until fairly recently in China, most people were not literate and had to memorize whatever they wanted to retain. This pervaded the culture in surprising ways. For example, an abacus is in many ways as much a means to facilitate numerical memory work as it is a primitive mechanical calculator. (Similarly. many Caucasians are astounded by those with a Jewish or Muslim heritage who can recite, from memory, long passages from their religious texts, although memorizing long passages of the Bible was once fashionable in North America. This was due partly to the lack of books and partly because it was seen as the best way of learning the material.)

These texts, once written down and published, first in China and then eventually throughout the world, served in the same way as the best of the traditional solo forms. In other words, these songs and solo forms were meant to be ways of practicing what you already knew how to do effectively, both by yourself or with another human being. Neither was meant to teach the basics.

I would recommend the translations that have appeared in recent years by the scholar Douglas Wile, as well as those by Dr. Yang Jwing-ming, Tim Cartmell, and Andrea Falk, as studying the taiji classics can be a fascinating side of the study of the Yang style.

Oh, and are you surprised that there are many controversies and arguments over whose translations are the best?

Losing Face

One of the more subtle cultural issues that can be important in a taiji class, especially if it is taught by an older Chinese teacher or if there are a lot of first-generation Chinese students, is the issue of "face."

It was and is sometimes still considered a terrible insult in Chinese culture to cause someone to publicly lose face. This can be done by something as simple as appearing to question or challenge the teacher in a group class. The person asking questions, perhaps in all innocence, has a two-edged sword to face in the sense that if he or she asks a stupid question, he or she may well lose face in relation to the other students as well as the teacher.

Conversely, if he or she asks an intelligent question that the teacher has trouble answering, then he or she has made the teacher lose face in front of the student body. In the old days in the Orient, causing the teacher to lose face in front of the other students might have gotten you a beating from him or his senior students in a rougher class, or expelled in a more civilized one.

In the old days, you didn't ask; you copied to the best of your ability or waited for the teacher to bring up the issues that troubled you. There are reports in Robert W. Smith's books on Cheng Man Ching saying that he asked questions about push-hands only twice in the time that he spent studying with Yang Cheng-fu and was injured both times by the very physical answers that he was given for his impertinence.

Of course, in a modern class, losing face is usually less of a physical issue for the student, but this cultural aspect of taiji training may help to explain why it used to be said that it took 10 years to become a good practitioner. If you can't ask questions because of the issue of face or get corrected in a group class setting because of the issue of face, it will be much harder to understand many of the details of practice and you'll have to struggle along to get it on your own unless eventually accepted into the inner circle of senior students.

In a more modern class, you don't have to worry about such issues as commonly as in the past, but some people still worry excessively about looking stupid by asking questions for which they assume that everyone else present will already have answers. However, a good teacher creates an atmosphere in which the students are not afraid to ask intelligent questions.

ETIQUETTE, ETHICS, AND OTHER UNFASHIONABLE CONCEPTS

There is an etiquette to visiting taiji classes or to studying with a particular teacher, and I'll outline some of the most important points for those unfamiliar with such issues.

As an Observer

- If you are going to a particular school to observe a class, then phone or e-mail ahead of time to say that you will be coming and why. When you arrive, tell whoever greets you at the door that you would like permission to observe a class and that you are just curious, or are shopping for a school, or whatever is appropriate.

- It's always a good idea to politely inquire about the teacher's experience and qualifications, especially if it is a commercial, public school, but older teachers (especially Chinese ones) who teach privately or out of their homes or public parks may interpret this as an insult.
- Don't get misunderstood by asking for a demonstration of skill from a teacher you have just met unless you smile sincerely first and make it clear that such is not just a thinly-veiled martial challenge. It was common enough (and still sometimes occurs) for a visitor to ask for a "lesson in push-hands," which really means, "Show me what you can do martially!"
- If you are observing a class, it is considered polite to leave only at the end of the class. If you must do otherwise, let whoever you have spoken to know ahead of time that you will be doing so. At the very least, try to leave in an unobtrusive manner and if possible catch the teacher's eye, smile and mouth a "thank you." Courtesy seems to be a dying art in modern society, but it costs nothing to be that way.
- If you watch a class with a friend, be quiet and don't talk needlessly to each other. Remember that if you laugh or make caustic comments, the teacher or some of his students may misinterpret your actions and ask that you leave—or worse.
- Never touch weapons on display, wander around the training area, or go into the changing rooms.

As a New Student

- If you aren't informed immediately, it is wise to learn what the instructor wants to be called while in class.

Although it has become famous in North America thanks to television and the movies, the title Sifu is rarely used in Northern China when addressing a teacher of martial arts, although it is used in that context in Southern China. A better title for a Chinese teacher of traditional martial arts is *Laoshi*, meaning, literally, "teacher," while the correct term for a teacher with more modern attitudes might be *Jiaolian*, which means "coach." By the way, some schools will insist that you use and learn some Chinese terminology for the training methods and forms as well as the ranking structure (if there is one). If you don't have an ear for language, then this can be one more challenge in your learning curve.

- Some schools have a very strict code of conduct while on the premises, while others are more relaxed. In general, modern taiji schools tend to be much more "laissez-faire" in such matters than schools in the Japanese or Korean traditions. In fact, more than one instructor whom I respect who has trained in China has told me that the atmosphere is usually quite relaxed and informal and that kowtowing, military-type discipline and uniforms are more often found in the classes run by Westerners than with the Chinese old-timers.
- On the other hand, in a traditional environment, it is quite often expected that you will provide money for gifts for teacher on special occasions, such as Chinese New Year or birthdays. This is not always done with tact. "I'm collecting money to buy teacher his birthday gift; your donation will be $25," was something I experienced often enough in different training environments. If the quality of instruction is good, you may have to live with this and other cultural peccadilloes to be able to continue to train there.

- In the end, common courtesy should rule and it is always best to treat your teacher, the senior students, and your peers with the respect required. One of the essential aspects of life is learning to get along with people on many levels. Shouldn't that be the first lesson learned in any style of self-defense?

Getting Martial Virtue

Martial ability (wugong) refers to physical training and experience in external or internal martial arts. It also implies a balanced approach to incorporating physical and "energetic" aspects to one's training. This is different from martial virtue (wude), which refers to a code of personal conduct that guides and restrains the practitioner when using his or her martial abilities outside the training hall.

Nowadays, wude is an often neglected aspect of modern taiji, although teachers often talk of using form practice or sitting or standing qigong as a means of meditation. However, little class time is usually devoted to such lofty aims.

This can be for practical reasons. For example, the teacher may not be an experienced practitioner of meditation, or may focus on teaching those who gravitate to the active life of martial training and is often the least likely to want to stand or sit quietly for any reasons as part of that training. There is no doubt that it is hard to understand why standing or sitting meditation can actually benefit your martial skills until you have experienced such training for yourself.

Conversely, a substantial proportion of modern beginners have some expectation that their teacher will be like the venerable chief monk on the old *Kung Fu* television series. They expect that the classes and the training will be exotic and mysterious, not just hard physical effort and the occasional bruise or injury. It is true that the martial artist was and still is often the subject of hero worship in the Orient.

There are many examples in Chinese popular fiction, going back decades—even centuries—of warrior ascetics whose kung fu skills were as highly developed as their social consciences. It is another question as to how often the real martial experts ever lived up to this lofty ideal, but the myths remain and do provide laudable theoretical role models—in fact, much better social role models than the overall atmosphere of bloodshed and revenge that tends to drive the kung fu cinema.

Those who choose to teach have a greater burden in some ways than those who are content to follow. Ideally, teaching a martial art should benefit the students on many levels, each according to his or her capacity and needs, and not just stroke the ego of the teacher or fill his pockets with money. One of my former instructors, Allan Weiss, often told me how his Chinese taiji instructor had described the most important aspect of teaching in his indifferent English as "having a good heart for the people."

Maybe it's because I am getting older and have so rarely come across an emphasis on ethics and etiquette in the taiji and Chinese martial arts schools that I have frequented, but I have grown to feel that it is essential to instill values in your training that are worthy of inspection from the perspective of any good religion or philosophy. May I suggest that the key concepts of a code of modern martial ethics might be respect, loyalty, honesty, humility, and integrity?

Respect

On a core level, you must respect both the art that you want to learn as well as your teacher, both as a person and as a teacher. If you already feel that you know as much as the person who is teaching you, it will be very difficult to understand the subtleties that often define the difference between a competent technician and a master practitioner.

You must also respect your training partners in class so that you approach each session as being a "learning experience" that must usually have some aspects of cooperation to be done safely and to the mutual benefit of all concerned. This is of particular importance when training with those who are more junior to you in terms of experience and skill.

Sadly, many people who approach the martial arts initially do so out of fear and their egos are tender in terms of being slighted or appearing stupid. A good teacher will not tolerate a student, senior or otherwise, who likes to "throw his weight around" and bully his juniors in class.

In the end, if you can't show respect for others in and out of your training, then it will be very difficult to get through life with any self respect and vice-versa. In a practical way, we get treated the way that we treat others.

Loyalty

In the old days, martial loyalty to a teacher was expected to be unconditional for the select few students. That role model literally assumed the role of an adoptive parent with the unquestioned obedience that this implied in Chinese culture. Such a concept is hard for Westerners to digest and has largely disappeared from modern North American schools, but is often still met in schools that have many first-generation Chinese students or a traditional approach to training.

Loyalty is a two-edged sword in the sense that practitioners are hardly liable to make the most of their training if they constantly hop from teacher to teacher or if they feel no sense of connection to what is being taught. However, it is equally true that a student must at the same time remain loyal to himself, his family, and society in general, as some disturbed or unscrupulous teachers will not hesitate to exploit obedience and respect from the students for financial, sexual, or egotistical reasons. It can be a fine balancing act to remain loyal both to your own needs and to those of the person teaching you.

Honesty

The teacher must be honest with the student and the student must be honest with the teacher and, perhaps the hardest of all, with himself or herself! As I suggested in an earlier chapter that you need to identify what you want from your training and reconcile those needs with what you can realistically achieve over the long term from your taijiquan—and communicate this to your teacher.

It is also important to realize that the teacher may have as much trouble as you do in identifying what he or she wants from being an instructor. Some do so for the money to be made from teaching commercially, some from a desire to be in the spotlight. Some teach from a genuine need to share whatever skills they may have.

These are all normal motives for teaching and, as long as the teacher is honest with the student and vice-versa and both are getting something from the relationship, then neither should have any real reason to complain about the relationship.

Humility

It's very difficult to learn anything if you already feel that you know it all. In particular, those students who already have some skills may well concentrate on trying to find the similarities between what they already think they know and with what they are presently studying. As I have said before, it is often more productive in understanding a new method or style to try and identify how it is different, rather than how it is similar to what you have done before.

It is perhaps even more important for the teacher to remain humble despite his or her technical skills and experience. It is perhaps the loss of this kind of "innocence" that keeps most instructors from fulfilling their real potentials as human beings and as practitioners and instructors. How can you learn more if you already feel that there is nothing left to learn from anyone else?

Integrity

This is something that has largely gone out of style in modern society and most people will no longer value the examples still to be found. For example, you find a wallet with a great deal of cash in it and go to the effort of returning it to its owner, your friends or family might look at you incredulously because you didn't accept a reward for its return (and more than a few will think you stupid for having taken it back in the first place).

Morality often seems to have little value in a consumer society whose heroes are politicians, media personalities, and the heads of large corporations, who seem to prosper because of their dubious or fraudulent practices.

This is not to say that you should try to become perfect or live like a mythic figure, but just stay true to whatever value system your parents raised you with. And, if they didn't raise you with a value system, it's never too late to learn.

Although it has nothing to do with martial training—or does it?—I recommend the advice of the Dalai Lama during a public address that he made on the subject of the millennium in the year 2000: "Follow the three Rs: respect for self, respect for others, responsibility for all your actions." Good advice for people in general and martial artists in particular!

FINAL THOUGHTS

Some experts will try to avoid discussing the traditional approach to qi and to some of the more esoteric training methods that seem old-fashioned, while others go to excess in terms of revering what came before—or what they imagine came before—while still others reduce everything to mechanical analogies in an attempt to appeal to the Western scientific approach. I think that there is room for all of these aspects in the serious study of taijiquan, especially for the student who is careful to maintain a sense of proportion and some common sense.

I won't pretend to understand the theories and controversies in modern science and physics beyond saying that, in my limited reading, the various experts seem to agree about as much as the various taiji experts do on various details. In the end, my only real problem with the Western approach is that it seems to persist in trying to understand the universe by dissecting and examining its various aspects in relative isolation.

Still, I have done much the same in this chapter, so I guess that I shouldn't fault others for demonstrating the same flaws!

ENDNOTES

1. The traditional Chinese approach to the human spine was that it didn't have a major folding or bending role and that the three major joints responsible for folding or bending were at the ankles, the knees, and the hips. The spine and skull were considered a unit in most ways and folding or bending except in subtle ways at the lower back and in the neck were no-nos!

2. Western boxing was popular with Chinese audiences in Shanghai in the 1920s and a few progressive martial arts teachers studied aspects of that system. Modern Sanda fighting in China incorporates Western boxing techniques as well.

Final Thoughts

If I have any last words of advice to share with those of you who are or who become serious about your training in the Yang style, it is that you should investigate a variety of teachers (a process which can take years) until you find one whose approach suits you both physically and emotionally. Having found this "priceless pearl," stick to him or her even if doing so means that you have to give up other styles that you may have practiced and enjoyed. It bears repeating that it is better, in the long run, to do a few things really well than to do a hundred things indifferently!

Similarly, the simple things in life are often the most meaningful in the long run. Don't neglect the forms or methods that seem basic in favor of those that are exotic or overly complex.

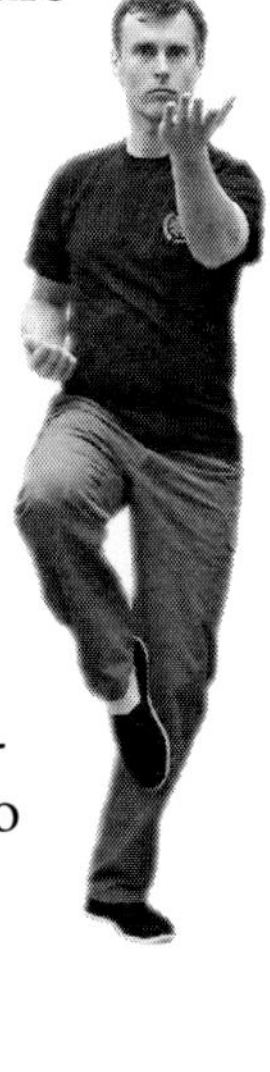

You have to have faith in yourself, your teachers, and the methods and forms that they practice or teach. Once lost, such faith is very difficult if not impossible to get back. However, don't be too arrogant in your faith in yourself and those who teach you, as this can easily lead to feeling that you are somehow superior to those who teach or practice differently from you.

You should learn, in martial terms, to "turn the other cheek," as this is almost always possible in real life unless you have the misfortune to live in a war zone. The world is already full of those who lash out in fear and anger. Shouldn't your training make you less fearful, less angry, and not just more martially skillful?

More and more, it seems to me that the real goal of taiji and internal martial arts training in general is to be a healthy, happy, and compassionate human being, and not just to become a peerless fighter.

In the end, there are no good reasons to get into a fight unless you have to defend yourself or a loved one against aggression, or you have a competitive nature and love martial sports

Conversely, there are many more good reasons to learn a competent martial expression of taijiquan:

- Building character through a healthy self-discipline
- Building, improving, and maintaining physical health, no matter what your age
- Learning how effective standing or moving meditation can be for improving emotional health
- Enjoying and exploring aspects of another culture without being blind to their imperfections
- Learning valid self-defense skills

If the world was a different, kinder place, then there would be no need for effective martial arts. Until that happy day, those with the will to do so can learn to find a balance of hard and soft through Yang-style taijiquan.

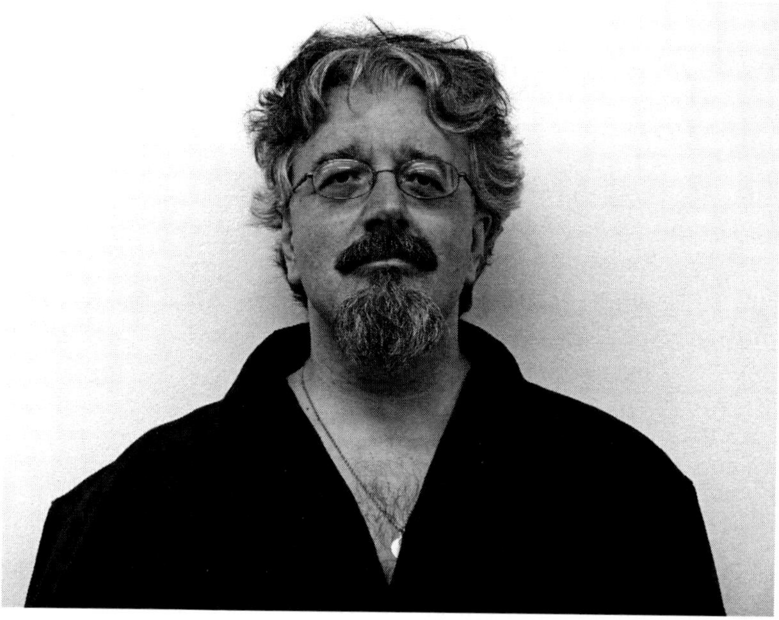

About the Author

After several years of lackluster attempts to learn karate, jujitsu, and Praying Mantis kung fu in the early 1970s, I began studying the Yang style in Ottawa in 1975 with a succession of instructors—the best of whom were Shirley and Steven Choi. By 1980, I was sure I knew it all. Then I met Allan Weiss, a senior student of the late Lee Shiu Pak in Montreal (Master Lee had studied in Shanghai with Chen Wei Ming, a senior student of Yang Cheng-fu). Allan soon shattered all my illusions about both my level of understanding of Yang style taiji and my martial expertise. After five years of studying with Allan, he certified me as an instructor in 1985.

For the next few years, I taught my own classes; studied Jeet Kune Do and Wing Chun Do as well as taijiquan, and wrote articles for a variety of martial arts magazines. I also traveled in Canada and the United States to do workshops and training camps with a variety of experts such as Eric Chew, Sam Masich, Yang Ywing Ming, Liang Shou Yu, William C.C. Chen, and Carol Mancuso. Each, in their own ways, helped me realize that I still didn't know as much as I had assumed.

I had been corresponding with Erle Montaigue since the late 1980s and invited him to Ottawa to do a workshop the first time that he toured North America in 1990. As a result of that experience, I decided to "start over" through his instructional videos and subsequent workshops that he gave in Ottawa and New Jersey. He eventually certified me to teach his approach to the Yang style (1992) and later his baguazhang curriculum (1994).

In recent years I have begun studying the Sun-style taijiquan as well as xingyiquan. Many years after my first Yang-style taiji class in the summer of 1975, I still don't have many answers relevant to taijiquan and the Chinese internal arts, but some of the questions are starting to make sense!

I have taught introductory courses at a variety of local community and fitness centers as well as running the Tai Chi Studio at the same location in downtown Ottawa since 1997. My first two books, *Tai Chi Chuan: The Martial Side* and *Power Taiji* (the latter co-written with Erle Montaigue), were published by Paladin Press in 1992 and 1995 respectively. A handbook on baguazhang for my students was self-published in 2004, followed by one on the Yang-style taijiquan in 2005.

Born in 1952, I live in Ottawa, Canada, with my wife, two sons, and a cute but annoying little cat named Willo.